Hand
Drug

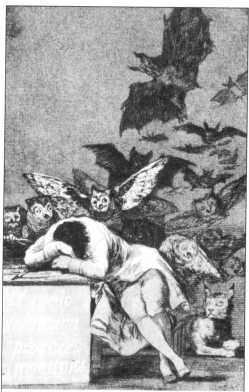

The Sleep of Reason Produces Monsters (Francisco Goya)

from the library of

Jeff Goldberg *M.D.*
8 - 95

compliments of
Scios Nova Inc.

Eskalith CR
(lithium carbonate)

Handbook of Psychiatric Drug Therapy

Third Edition

Steven E. Hyman, M.D.

Associate Professor of Psychiatry and Neuroscience, Harvard Medical School; Director of Psychiatry Research, Massachusetts General Hospital, Boston, Massachusetts

George W. Arana, M.D.

Professor of Psychiatry, Medical University of South Carolina College of Medicine; Medical Director and Associate Dean, Medical University of South Carolina Medical Center, Charleston, South Carolina

Jerrold F. Rosenbaum, M.D.

Associate Professor of Psychiatry, Harvard Medical School; Director, Outpatient Psychiatry, Massachusetts General Hospital, Boston, Massachusetts

Little, Brown and Company
Boston   New York   Toronto   London

Library of Congress Cataloging-in-Publication Data
Hyman, Steven E.
    Handbook of psychiatric drug therapy / Steven E. Hyman, George W.
Arana, Jerrold F. Rosenbaum.—3rd ed.
        p.   cm.
    Arana's name appears first on second edition.
    Includes bibliographical references and index.
    ISBN 0-316-04946-8
    1. Mental illness—Chemotherapy—Handbooks, manuals, etc.
2. Psychopharmacology—Handbooks, manuals, etc.   I. Arana, George
W.   II. Rosenbaum, J. F. (Jerrold F.)   III. Title.
    [DNLM: 1. Mental Disorders—drug therapy.   2. Psychotropic Drugs—
pharmacology.   WM 402 H996y 1995]
RC483.A73   1995
616.89'18—dc20
DNLM/DLC
for Library of Congress   95-1489
                                                                    CIP

Printed in the United States of America
RRD-VA

Editorial: Nancy Megley, Richard Wilcox
Copyeditor: Debra Corman
Indexer: Nancy Newman
Production Supervisor/Designer: Michael A. Granger

To Barbara, Emily, Julia, Betsy,
Isabel, Julia, Ashley, Lidia, Jed, Eliza, and Blake

Contents

Disease-Specific Table of Contents

This table provides the reader with easy access to major places in the book that discuss the indications for medications in specific disorders or clinical situations. The major chapters in which a disorder is discussed are given in bold. This table does not refer to every citation; that purpose is served by the index.

Preface

This handbook is a practical guide to the use of the various categories of modern psychiatric drugs. It is written in a way that should be useful for psychiatrists but easily accessible to generalists and to other health professionals who are involved in the management of patients with psychiatric disorders. We have avoided the encyclopedic approach and focused on the major classes of drugs used in clinical practice. In the interest of brevity and practicality, we have excluded those agents whose use is primarily of historic interest (e.g., some of the older sedative-hypnotics). We have attempted to delineate what is known on the basis of controlled clinical trials, but in the areas where there is little systematic evidence to guide clinical practice, we have tried not to allow pedantry to interfere with practicality and clinical need.

S.E.H.
G.W.A.
J.F.R.

Handbook of Psychiatric Drug Therapy

1

Introduction to Psychopharmacology

The practice of psychopharmacology can be extremely challenging. Psychiatric disorders frequently have unpredictable courses, complicating comorbid psychiatric or medical disorders are common, and symptoms of psychiatric disorders may interfere with compliance (e.g., denial of illness in mania, suspiciousness in many psychotic disorders, and a pattern of interpersonal turmoil in certain personality disorders that does not spare caregivers). Additionally, medications are not fully effective in many patients. Although in some illnesses, such as major depression, bipolar disorder, and panic disorder, available therapies help the majority of patients, many patients respond only incompletely, and a substantial minority prove treatment refractory. For other disorders, such as schizophrenia, the current treatments are only palliative, leaving the patient with many disabling symptoms. It takes great skill for the practitioner to maintain the right balance between pharmacologic and psychological approaches to therapy. Skilled use of the psychiatric drugs currently available can result in good outcomes for many patients who would otherwise suffer severe morbidity or even death.

Although pharmacologic interventions are the most effective treatments for many psychiatric disorders (e.g., bipolar disorder, panic attacks, and major depression), cognitive and behavior therapy, family therapy, and psychodynamic psychotherapy should also be initiated if indicated. For many patients, the benefits of medical treatment and psychotherapy are additive or synergistic. For example, some patients who have panic disorder with agoraphobia may recover from their panic attacks with drug therapy but remain disabled by agoraphobia unless they participate in behavior therapy. Major depression responds well to pharmacotherapy, but many patients are optimally treated when medication and psychotherapy are combined to treat all aspects of their problem. On the other hand, there are situations, such as acute mania, in which psychotherapy might be counterproductive, worsening the acute symptoms.

In general, an ideological preference for either pharmacologic or psychosocial treatment, as opposed to reliance on the best available information derived from controlled studies, has no place in successful psychiatric practice. An ideological preference for one form of treatment over another, which may be caricatured as "Here is the treatment, now tell me the problem," serves patients' needs poorly. The standard of care for psychiatric disorders requires a careful diagnostic assessment prior to the introduction of therapy, and the therapy chosen must have documented efficacy for the patient's condition. This standard leaves much room for clinical judgment. The clinician must recognize that available controlled studies are an incomplete guide to actual clinical situations. Subjects eligible for clinical studies are a small subset of patients requiring treatment. They are typically relatively young, on no other medications, lacking serious comorbidity, and willing to be on a placebo for several weeks. Furthermore, clinical research trials that fully establish efficacy often lag behind clinical observation and practice by several years.

A case in point is the International Psychopharmacology Algorithm Project, where clinician researchers met to draft decision trees to provide prescribing practices for psychiatric disorders. From the outset it was clear that solid scientific data were barely available beyond the first node of the algorithm. Few existing studies addressed the approach to initial treatment failures, poor responders, or those discontinuing treatment due to side effects. Moreover, for panic disorder, for example, the most extensive data available supported the use of imipramine as the initial treatment of choice. The consensus among the assembled experts, however, was that selective serotonin reuptake inhibitors were their clinical choice, despite the absence of completed controlled trials at that time. The panel agreed to construct the algorithm to reflect their actual preferred clinical choices but qualified their choices with descriptions indicating the quality of available supporting evidence: A for replicated controlled studies, B for open trials and pilot studies, and C for clinical observations and anecdotes. This compromise is consistent with the philosophy of this book—to present state-of-the-art clinical psychopharmacology emphasizing clinical practice as informed by clinical science.

In the spirit of practicality, we offer certain principles that have guided our treatment of major psychiatric illnesses and that we believe have general merit in psychiatric drug therapy.

BEFORE INITIATING MEDICATIONS

1. Before prescribing psychotropic medication, it is important to be clear as to the diagnosis. If the diagnosis is unsure, a clear set of diagnostic hypotheses should be established, and a systematic approach to clarifying the diagnosis should be outlined. For example, depressive, psychotic, or catatonic states may result from medical or psychiatric illness or from drug abuse, or they may represent an adverse reaction to antipsychotic drugs.

2. Before prescribing psychotropic medications, it is important to be aware of medical problems or drug interactions that could (a) be responsible for the patient's psychiatric symptoms, (b) increase the toxicity of prescribed drugs (e.g., diuretics or nonsteroidal anti-inflammatory agents may increase lithium levels), or (c) decrease the effectiveness of the planned therapy (e.g., anticonvulsants hasten the metabolism of tricyclic antidepressants).

3. Be aware of the possibility of alcohol or drug abuse, which might confound treatment. It is recommended that patients first be detoxified from alcohol or drugs rather than attempting treatment of a presumed psychiatric disorder (e.g., depression) during ongoing substance abuse.

4. Before prescribing a psychiatric medication, it is imperative to identify **target symptoms** (e.g., sleep disturbance, panic attacks, or hallucinations) that can be followed during the course of therapy to monitor the success of treatment. It is also important to monitor changes in the patient's quality of life (e.g., satisfaction with home and family life, functioning at work, and overall sense of well-being). An alternative for patients who cannot report their own symptoms (e.g., demented or psychotic patients) is to ask the patient's family to rate behavior (e.g., a simple daily rating on a scale of 1–10 points). The use of identified target symptoms and quality of life assessment is especially important when the medication is being given as an **empirical trial** in a patient whose diagnosis is unclear.

5. Principles of optimal drug selection are presented throughout this manual. However, if a medication was previously effective and very well tolerated by a patient, it is a reasonable clinical judgment

to use that medication again even if newer drugs are now available for the patient's condition.

6. When there is doubt about the correct diagnosis or therapy, consultation should be sought. The clinician's response to the consultant's recommendations (including agreement or disagreement) should be documented.

ADMINISTRATION OF MEDICATIONS

1. Once a drug is chosen, **administer a full trial with adequate doses and duration of treatment** so that if the target symptoms do not improve, there will be no need to return to that agent. (Inadequate dosing and duration are the main reasons for failure of antidepressant trials in well-diagnosed patients.)

2. Be aware of side effects, and warn patients in advance if appropriate (e.g., about sedation early in the course of daytime benzodiazepine use, or dry mouth or blurred vision with tricyclic antidepressants). Develop a clear idea of which toxicities require reassurance (e.g., dry mouth), treatment (e.g., neuroleptic-induced parkinsonism), or drug discontinuation (e.g., lithium-induced interstitial nephritis). Examine patients when appropriate (e.g., for rigidity or oral dyskinesia). Recall that the side effects of some psychotropic agents may mimic symptoms of the disorder being treated (e.g., neuroleptic-induced akathisia may present as agitation; neuroleptic-induced akinesia may be indistinguishable from catatonia due to the illness).

3. When possible, keep regimens simple both to improve compliance and to avoid additive toxicity. Compliance is often enhanced if regimens and dosing schedules are kept simple (e.g., lithium qd or bid instead of tid or qid), if patients are engaged in a dialogue about the time course of expected improvement, and if complaints about side effects are taken seriously. Patients who are psychotic, demented, or retarded may need careful supervision from family to maintain compliance.

4. Readjust the dosage of medication to determine the lowest effective dose for the particular stage of the patient's illness because, for psychotic disorders in particular, dosage requirements often change over time. For example, in schizophrenia, the dosage of antipsychotic medication that is needed to treat acute exacerbations is generally higher than for long-term maintenance.

5. In the elderly, it is prudent to initiate treatment with lower doses of medication. Dosage changes should be less frequent in the elderly than in younger patients because the time required for drugs to achieve steady state levels is often prolonged.

6. Follow-up care includes evaluating efficacy of treatment; monitoring and managing side effects, treatment-relevant intercurrent life events, and comorbid medical and psychiatric conditions; obtaining and evaluating appropriate laboratory data; and when necessary, planning changes in the treatment regimen. These elements of care require the budgeting of adequate time. The authors generally budget 15–30 minutes for a follow-up visit with a relatively stable patient.

DISCONTINUATION OF MEDICATIONS

1. All too often ineffective medications are continued indefinitely and multiple medications accumulate in the patient's regimen, leading to unnecessary costs and side effects. Adjunctive and combina-

tion therapies may be appropriate for certain conditions; however, when medications no longer prove useful to the treatment regimen, it is critical to discontinue them. It may be difficult to determine that a medication has failed unless the physician has kept track of objective target symptoms from the beginning of the trial.

2. Even after apparent therapeutic success, criteria for discontinuation of psychotropic drugs in most clinical situations are ill-defined. When discontinuing psychotropic medications, it is best to taper dosages slowly, which can help prevent rebound or withdrawal symptoms. Because they have different therapeutic implications, it is important to distinguish among temporary symptom **rebound** (as frequently occurs after discontinuing short-acting benzodiazepines), which is brief and transient, but often severe; **recurrence** of the disorder, in which original symptoms return long-term; and **withdrawal**, in which new symptoms characteristic of withdrawal from the particular drug appear. In general, conditions that have been chronic before treatment, recurrent, or have emerged late in life are more likely to require long-term maintenance treatment.

OTHER ISSUES IN PSYCHOPHARMACOLOGY

1. To optimize clinical management of complicated illnesses, it is important to **document** observations of the patient (including mental status at baseline and changes with treatment), clinical reasoning, and side effects. Particular attention should be given to documenting risk of suicide or violence and risk of serious side effects such as tardive dyskinesia. It is also important for the record to indicate that the patient understands the reason for treatment, its risks and benefits, alternative treatments, and the risks of no treatment. If the competence of the patient to make his or her own decisions fluctuates or is questionable, the clinician should obtain the patient's permission to include the family in important treatment decisions. If the patient is clearly not competent to make decisions, a formal legal mechanism for substituted judgment must be used.

2. Many of the drugs discussed in this book have not been approved by the Food and Drug Administration for the particular indication discussed (e.g., beta-adrenergic blockers or anticonvulsants for psychiatric disorders in general or fluoxetine for panic disorder). However, a physician is free to choose any approved drug for nonapproved indications. The record should reflect the basis for this clinical decision, which ideally should reflect appreciation and understanding of the available evidence.

3. The cost of therapeutic drugs is an important issue in treatment selection. For clinicians, the principle guiding drug choice is "cost-effectiveness." The cheapest drug may be the least cost-effective if suboptimal clinical outcome, diminished quality of life, and costs due to side effects offset the initial savings. If compliance is enhanced and relapse diminished, and if safety is enhanced, thus reducing the cost of follow-up, an initially more costly drug may be the most cost-effective choice. Thus a narrow focus on drug costs of the formulary alone is inadequate. On the other hand, where drugs are equally safe and effective, cost is a valid basis for selection.

Antipsychotic Drugs

Antipsychotic drugs have been in clinical use since the 1950s, when chlorpromazine, a phenothiazine derivative, was synthesized in France. Although developed as a potential antihistamine, chlorpromazine was noted to have potent psychotropic properties in clinical trials. It was first used as a preanesthetic agent and within 2 years was found to be effective in the treatment of psychotic patients.

Although usually referred to as antipsychotic drugs, the drugs in this group have other therapeutic usages (e.g., as antiemetics, preanesthetics, and in palliation of some movement disorders). The term *neuroleptic* (meaning causing a neurologic disorder) has also been applied to the standard compounds in this class because of the profound extrapyramidal motor side effects (EPS) they may produce. These motor effects markedly complicate the use of antipsychotic drugs. An exception is the antipsychotic drug clozapine, which has relatively few and mild effects on the motor system (although it does have other serious side effects). A widely used terminology has developed to distinguish those antipsychotic drugs that have a high likelihood of producing EPS from those that do not. The antipsychotic drugs that produce EPS are usually called typical antipsychotic drugs. These drugs are high-affinity antagonists of D_2 dopamine receptors. In contrast, clozapine is often called an atypical antipsychotic drug. As noted, clozapine has substantially less tendency to produce EPS; this likely reflects the fact that it has a lower (albeit still significant) affinity for D_2 dopamine receptors relative to the typical antipsychotic drugs. Despite manufacturer claims, all of the antipsychotic drugs approved for use in the United States, except for clozapine, should be classified as typical antipsychotics, although there is no hard and fast demarcation. Some clinicians might classify the recently approved drug risperidone as atypical, but in fact it does cause EPS, especially in higher doses. The search for novel, truly atypical antipsychotic drugs that are less toxic than clozapine is a matter of intense research at the present time.

The antipsychotic drugs are the cornerstone of treatment for a wide variety of psychotic disorders; nonetheless their side effects may be severe, and some of the side effects of typical antipsychotic drugs (e.g., akathisia or akinesia) can mimic or exacerbate the symptoms for which the drugs were originally prescribed. Long-term use of these drugs can result in the syndrome of tardive dyskinesia (TD), which produces long-standing or permanent abnormal involuntary movements. Thus, despite the low risk of lethal toxicity from overdose of antipsychotic drugs (making them much safer in this regard than the tricyclic antidepressants or lithium), their optimal use is difficult.

CHEMISTRY

Although all antipsychotic agents available in the United States except for clozapine are high-affinity D_2 dopamine receptor antagonists, they vary considerably in chemical structure. **Phenothiazines**, the first chemical class of antipsychotic drugs developed, are tricyclic molecules. Three subtypes of phenothiazines are available: (1) aliphatics, (2) piperidines, and (3) piperazines. These subtypes differ chemically depending on the substituent on a ring-

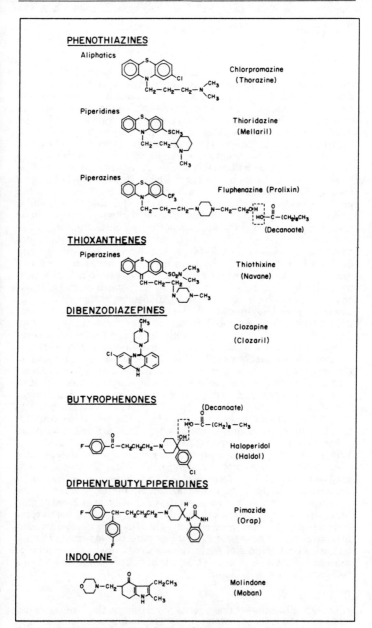

Fig. 2-1. Chemical structures of selected antipsychotic drugs.

nitrogen (Fig. 2-1). Although definitive structure-activity relationships for these drugs are not known, some observations can be made about how these substitutions affect drug action. Those phenothiazines with **aliphatic** side chains (e.g., chlorpromazine) tend to be low-potency compounds (i.e., higher doses are needed to achieve therapeutic effectiveness). **Piperidine** substitutions impart anticholinergic properties and a lower incidence of extrapyramidal symptoms (e.g., thioridazine, mesoridazine). **Piperazine** phenothiazines (e.g., perphenazine, trifluoperazine, fluphenazine) are among the most potent antipsychotic drugs.

The **thioxanthene** class of antipsychotic drugs is chemically similar to the phenothiazines. The **butyrophenones** represent a class of extremely potent antipsychotic drugs. Of these, only haloperidol is currently approved for psychiatric use in the United States. Droperidol, a shorter-acting butyrophenone, is approved for use as a preanesthetic agent.

Several other compounds of varied chemical structures have been approved for the treatment of psychotic and other illnesses in the United States. Pimozide, a **diphenylbutylpiperidine** approved for Gilles de la Tourette syndrome, is also a potent antipsychotic drug that has a very long half-life (several days). Other heterocyclic compounds known to have antipsychotic efficacy include the indoles, represented by a **dihydroindolone**, molindone. Also, there are compounds closely resembling the tricyclic antidepressants with a seven-member central ring and a piperazine substitution called **dibenzodiazepines**; this class of antipsychotic drugs is represented by the typical antipsychotic drug, loxapine, and by the atypical drug, clozapine. Recently risperidone, a **benzisoxazole** derivative that combines high affinity for D_2 dopamine receptors and 5-HT$_2$ serotonin receptors, has been introduced as an antipsychotic drug.

PHARMACOLOGY

Potency Versus Efficacy

The basic pharmacologic distinction between potency and efficacy is helpful to an understanding of the antipsychotic drugs. **Efficacy** refers to the maximal therapeutic effect that can be achieved by a drug, while **potency** describes the amount of the drug needed to achieve that maximum effect. All of the typical antipsychotic drugs are equivalent in efficacy. Thus at an optimal dosage, which differs for each drug (Table 2-1), each of these agents has been found to be equally effective in treating psychotic disorders. Clozapine is the only well-established exception. A trial conducted in patients with schizophrenia who had been unresponsive to at least two different antipsychotic drugs found significant improvement in 30% of 126 patients treated with clozapine for 6 weeks compared with only 5% of 141 patients treated with chlorpromazine (Kane et al., 1988). Clinical experience has confirmed the results of this well-designed trial; that is, clozapine may effectively treat patients who do not respond to other antipsychotic drugs. Initial hope that risperidone might also have enhanced efficacy is still under investigation at the time of this writing. While the standard or typical antipsychotic drugs have similar efficacies, they differ markedly in potency (i.e., the dosage needed to obtain the maximum therapeutic effect). The least potent drugs, such as chlorpromazine, may require a 50-fold higher dosage than the most potent drugs, such as haloperidol or fluphenazine.

Table 2-1. Antipsychotic drugs: potencies and side effect profiles

Drug	Approximate dose equivalent (mg)	Sedative effect	Hypotensive effect	Anticholinergic effect	Extrapyramidal effect
Phenothiazines					
Aliphatic					
Chlorpromazine (Thorazine)	100	High	High	Medium	Low
Piperidines					
Mesoridazine (Serentil)	50	Medium	Medium	Medium	Medium
Thioridazine (Mellaril)	95	High	High	High	Low
Piperazines					
Fluphenazine (Prolixin, Permitil)	2	Medium	Low	Low	High
Perphenazine (Trilafon)	8	Low	Low	Low	High
Trifluoperazine (Stelazine)	5	Medium	Low	Low	High
Thioxanthene					
Thiothixene (Navane)	5	Low	Low	Low	High
Dibenzodiazepines					
Loxapine (Loxitane, Daxolin)	10	Medium	Medium	Medium	High
Clozapine (Clozaril)	100	High	High	High	Very low
Benzisoxazole					
Risperidone (Risperdal)	1–2	Low	Medium	Low	Low
Butyrophenones					
Droperidol (Inapsine—injection only)	1	Low	Low	Low	High
Haloperidol (Haldol)	2	Low	Low	Low	High
Indolone					
Molindone (Moban)	10	Medium	Low	Medium	High
Diphenylbutylpiperidine					
Pimozide (Orap)	1	Low	Low	Low	High

A useful generalization about the antipsychotic drugs (excluding risperidone) is that those with low potency tend to be more sedating, more anticholinergic, and cause more postural hypotension than the high-potency drugs. The high-potency drugs tend to cause more extrapyramidal symptoms. Risperidone may be an exception to this rule, representing a high-potency antipsychotic drug that may have a milder profile of EPS.

Absorption and Distribution

Antipsychotic drugs are available for both oral and parenteral use, although not all drugs are available in both forms (Table 2-2). Pharmacokinetics are well understood only for a few of the drugs, especially chlorpromazine, thioridazine, and haloperidol. Taken orally, the drugs are absorbed adequately, although somewhat variably. Food or antacids may decrease absorption. Liquid preparations are absorbed more rapidly and reliably than tablets. There is a marked first-pass effect through the liver with oral administration (i.e., a high percentage of the drug is metabolized as it passes through the hepatic portal circulation). The peak effect of an oral dose generally occurs within 2–4 hours.

Parenterally administered antipsychotics are rapidly and reliably absorbed. Drug effect is usually apparent within 15–20 minutes after intramuscular injection, with peak effect occurring within 30–60 minutes. With intravenous administration, some drug effect is apparent within minutes, and peak effect occurs within 20–30 minutes. (Intravenous administration of antipsychotic drugs has not been approved by the Food and Drug Administration [FDA] except for droperidol.) Since parenteral administration bypasses the first pass through the portal circulation, it results in a significantly higher serum level than equivalent oral dosages.

Antipsychotic drugs are generally highly protein-bound (85–90%). Clinicians should therefore be cautious when concomitantly treating with other medications that are highly protein-bound (e.g., warfarin, digoxin) because displacement and competition for these binding sites could alter effective concentrations of both antipsychotics and other drugs. Antipsychotics are also highly lipophilic; thus, they readily cross the blood-brain barrier and attain high concentrations in the brain. Indeed, concentrations in the brain appear to be greater than those in blood. Given their high degree of protein and tissue binding, these drugs are not removed efficiently by dialysis.

Metabolism and Elimination

Many antipsychotic drugs are metabolized in the liver to demethylated and hydroxylated forms. These are more water-soluble than the parent compounds and thus more readily excreted by the kidneys. The hydroxylated metabolites often are further metabolized by conjugation with glucuronic acid. Many of the hydroxyl and desmethyl metabolites of phenothiazines are active as dopamine receptor antagonists. The hydroxyl metabolite of the butyrophenone antipsychotic drug haloperidol (hydroxyhaloperidol) does not appear to be active. Much is unknown about the metabolites of other chemical classes of antipsychotics.

The elimination **half-life** of most of the antipsychotic drugs is 18–40 hours, but numerous factors, such as genetically determined metabolic rates, age, and the coadministration of other hepatically

Table 2-2. Available preparations of antipsychotic drugs

Drug	Tablets (mg)	Capsules (mg)	Sustained-release forms (mg)	Liquid concentrate[a]	Liquid suspension[a] or elixir	Syrup[a] (mg/5 ml)	Injection[b]
Phenothiazines							
Aliphatics							
Chlorpromazine (Thorazine, generics)	10, 25, 50, 100, 200		30, 75, 150, 200, 300	30 mg/ml, 100 mg/ml		10 mg/5 ml	25 mg/ml, 10 mg/ml
Piperidines							
Mesoridazine (Serentil)	10, 25, 50, 100			25 mg/ml			25 mg/ml
Thioridazine (Mellaril, generics)	10, 15, 25, 50, 100, 150, 200			30 mg/ml, 100 mg/ml	25 mg/5 ml, 100 mg/5 ml		
Piperazines							
Fluphenazine HCl (Prolixin, Permitil, generics)	1, 2.5, 5, 10			5 mg/ml	0.5 mg/1 ml, 2.5 mg/5 ml		2.5 mg/ml
Fluphenazine enanthate, decanoate (Prolixin)							25 mg/ml
Perphenazine (Trilafon, generics)	2, 4, 8, 16			16 mg/5 ml			5 mg/ml
Trifluoperazine (Stelazine, generics)	1, 2, 5, 10			10 mg/ml			2 mg/ml
Thioxanthene							
Thiothixene (Navane, generics)		1, 2, 5, 10, 20		5 mg/ml			2 mg/ml, 5 mg/ml

	Tablets (mg)	Liquid[a]	Parenteral[b]
Dibenzodiazepines			
Loxapine (Loxitane, generics)	5, 10, 25, 50	25 mg/ml	50 mg/ml
Clozapine (Clozaril)	25, 100		
Benzisoxazole			
Risperidone (Risperdal)	1, 2, 3, 4		
Butyrophenone			
Haloperidol (Haldol, generics)	0.5, 1, 2, 5, 10, 20	2 mg/ml	5 mg/ml
Haloperidol decanoate (Haldol)			50 mg/ml, 100 mg/ml
Indolone			
Molindone (Moban)	5, 10, 25, 50, 100	20 mg/ml	
Diphenylbutylpiperidine			
Pimozide (Orap)	2		

[a] Liquid form for oral use.
[b] Parenteral form, which is packaged in either a vial or ampule.

metabolized drugs, affect the half-life to such a degree that plasma levels may vary among individuals by 10- to 20-fold.

Long-Acting Preparations

Long-acting preparations of antipsychotic drugs in which the active drug is esterified to a lipid side chain are available. The drug is given as an intramuscular injection in an oily vehicle that slows absorption. The only depot preparations currently available in the United States are the decanoate ester of fluphenazine and the decanoate ester of haloperidol. Fluphenazine decanoate has a half-life of 7–10 days, allowing administration approximately every 2 weeks. Haloperidol decanoate has a longer half-life, allowing dosing intervals of 3–6 weeks, depending on the individual.

Blood Levels

Given the marked interindividual differences in plasma levels produced by a given oral dose and the concerns about the consequences of noncompliance among psychotic patients, it would be useful to have some objective measure of drug level to aid in optimizing efficacy and clinical improvement. Specifically, it has been hoped that a range of therapeutic blood levels could be determined for the various antipsychotic drugs. Unfortunately, the measurement of blood levels by various chromatographic techniques and mass spectroscopy has not correlated well with clinical response. This problem reflects, at least partly, the presence of many active metabolites. Some antipsychotic drugs have so many active metabolites (e.g., thioridazine) that measurement to assess dose-response relationships is impractical. At present, haloperidol blood levels as determined by either high-performance liquid chromatography or gas-liquid chromatography have shown promise. Haloperidol has one metabolite, hydroxyhaloperidol, which was thought to have weak antipsychotic activity, but recent data suggest that it has little or no activity. There is evidence that haloperidol levels greater than 5–10 ng/ml may correspond with clinical antipsychotic effects. At present, except for haloperidol, serum levels for antipsychotic drugs are probably more misleading clinically than they are useful because the putative "therapeutic" range reported for each drug has not been convincingly shown to correlate with clinical improvement. Thus, clinical observation and documentation of specific symptom changes over time remain the mainstays of assessment of drug efficacy.

MECHANISM OF ACTION

The major action of antipsychotic drugs in the nervous system is to block receptors for the neurotransmitter dopamine. However, the therapeutic mechanism of action of antipsychotic drugs is only partly understood. The typical (e.g., haloperidol-like) antipsychotic drugs are all potent antagonists of D_2 dopamine receptors. However, two novel D_2-like dopamine receptors have recently been discovered by molecular cloning. These receptors are currently called the D_3 and D_4 dopamine receptors, but it is possible that a change in nomenclature will prove necessary. All of the typical antipsychotic drugs also block D_3 and D_4 dopamine receptors. The atypical antipsychotic drug clozapine differs from all other antipsychotic drugs in clinical use in that it is a relatively weak D_2 receptor antagonist, which may explain why it does not cause significant extrapyramidal side effects and explains why it does not increase prolactin levels. More striking, however, is that unlike the other antipsychotic drugs, clozapine has a 10-fold higher affinity for the D_4 than for the D_2 dopamine receptor. Combined with the evidence that clozapine may exhibit unique clinical efficacy in schizophrenia, this observation has called into question a necessary role for D_2 receptor antagonism in antipsychotic drug action and has raised the possibility that the D_4 receptor may also be a significant therapeutic target.

Clozapine, however, also interacts with many other neurotransmitter receptors, including D_1 and D_3 dopamine, 5-HT$_{2C}$ serotonin, muscarinic cholinergic, and alpha$_1$-adrenergic receptors. This makes it difficult to argue that any single effect of the drug is responsible for its clinical properties. Indeed the recently introduced antipsychotic drug risperidone combines high affinity for D_2 dopamine receptors (like haloperidol) with high affinity for 5-HT$_{2C}$ serotonin receptors (like clozapine) on the hypothesis that antagonist effects at serotonin 5-HT$_{2C}$ receptors may diminish extrapyramidal side effects. Clinically, risperidone does appear to have less tendency to cause extrapyramidal side effects than equipotent doses of haloperidol, but early experience suggests that it may not have the unique efficacy of clozapine in treatment-refractory schizophrenic patients.

It is believed that the therapeutic actions of antipsychotic drugs are exerted via the mesolimbic and mesocortical dopamine projections in the brain (Fig. 2-2). Blockade of dopamine and other receptors elsewhere in the brain is responsible for some other useful effects of antipsychotic drugs—for example, dopamine blockade in the chemotrigger zone of the medulla makes these drugs potent antiemetics—but also for their serious side effects. Blockade of D_2 receptors in the striatum is responsible for the extrapyramidal effects of the typical antipsychotic drugs.

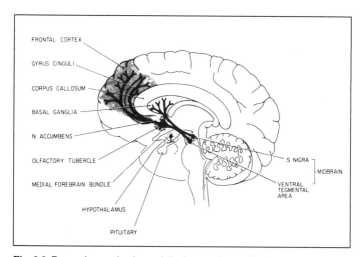

Fig. 2-2. Dopamine projections of the human brain. Cells in the substantia nigra project to the basal ganglia; cells in the ventral tegmental area of the midbrain project to frontal cortex and limbic areas. Hypothalamic dopamine neurons project to the pituitary.

In addition to these midbrain dopamine systems, there is a dopamine projection in the tuberoinfundibular system of the hypothalamus. In this system, dopamine acts as an inhibitor of the synthesis and release of prolactin by pituitary lactotrophs. By antagonizing dopamine in this system, antipsychotic drugs often produce hyperprolactinemia.

The full therapeutic effects of antipsychotic drugs take weeks to appear (similar to the antidepressants) and are far slower than the time required to block dopamine receptors or, in most cases, to achieve steady state plasma levels of the drug. Similarly, behavioral effects in patients can last long after serum levels are no longer detectable. Such observations suggest that the therapeutic response to antipsychotic drugs is a secondary or adaptive response to dopamine receptor blockade with a time course characterized by slower onset and offset than would be predicted simply by serum or even brain levels. (Human brain levels may now be inferred experimentally from positron emission tomography.) It must also be recognized that some initially responsive patients relapse even with apparently adequate serum levels of drug, suggesting that other types of adaptations may occur in the brain reflecting such factors as primary alterations in the disease process, changes in the psychosocial circumstances of the patient's life, intercurrent psychiatric or physical illness, or drug tolerance. The therapeutically relevant delayed-onset neurobiologic effects of antipsychotic drugs remain unknown.

In addition to their effects on dopamine receptors, antipsychotic drugs may cause side effects by binding to a variety of other neurotransmitter receptors. For example, low-potency antipsychotic drugs are potent antagonists of muscarinic cholinergic receptors with a relative affinity of thioridazine > chlorpromazine > mesoridazine. (Recall that mesoridazine is a metabolite of thioridazine as well as being marketed as an antipsychotic in its own right.) Clozapine also has substantial anticholinergic potency. As a result, these drugs produce side effects such as dry mouth and constipation. Postural hypotension is produced by antagonism of alpha$_1$-adrenergic receptors. Antipsychotic drugs with substantial affinity for this receptor are mesoridazine > chlorpromazine > thioridazine. Sedation appears to result from antagonism of several neurotransmitter receptors, including alpha$_1$-adrenergic, muscarinic, and histamine H_1 receptors. Because of substantial affinity for these receptor types, low-potency antipsychotics, such as chlorpromazine and thioridazine, are sedating. Additionally, many antipsychotic drugs block certain calcium channels on neurons, cardiac muscle, and smooth muscle. Thioridazine and pimozide are particularly potent calcium channel blockers, which may explain their cardiac toxicity (prolongation of the QTc interval with risk of torsades de pointes ventricular tachycardia). It has been hypothesized that the side effect of retrograde ejaculation caused by thioridazine is also due to its calcium antagonist properties.

INDICATIONS

Overview

Occasionally antipsychotic drugs have been referred to as antischizophrenic drugs but they are effective in a wide variety of disorders (Table 2-3). Indeed, given their broad spectrum of effectiveness, a patient's response to these agents is not helpful in making a diagnosis (e.g., a history of response is not diagnostic of schizophrenia). In addition to their antipsychotic action, these drugs have sedating effects in some patients. Because of their extrapyramidal effects and especially the risk of TD, the long-term use of typical antipsychotic drugs must generally be limited to treatment of psychoses and refractory bipolar disorder. Although clozapine does not appear to cause EPS or TD, its own serious side effects, and particularly the risk of agranulocytosis, requiring weekly blood drawing, limit its utility.

In addition to their use in psychiatric disorders, most antipsychotics are potent antiemetics, and many of them (e.g., prochlorperazine) are marketed for that indication. In addition, the short-acting, extremely potent butyrophenone droperidol is used as a preanesthetic drug but can also be useful in the treatment of acute psychoses. Finally, these drugs, by virtue of their dopamine receptor antagonism, are used to control severe choreoathetoid movements arising in such conditions as Huntington's disease or hemiballismus.

Schizophrenia

Schizophrenia probably represents a heterogeneous group of disorders with certain core clinical features. It is a chronic illness in which psychotic symptoms are prominent (e.g., hallucinations, delusions, ideas of reference, and/or thought disorder). Although the course may be punctuated by acute exacerbations followed by periods of less florid psychosis, the course of this illness over years involves deterioration of function and generally an inability to maintain an active and productive life.

Table 2-3. **Indications for use of antipsychotic drugs**

Short-term use (≤ 3 mos)
Effective
    Exacerbations of schizophrenia
    Acute mania
    Depression with psychotic features (combined with antidepressant)
    Other acute psychoses (e.g., schizophreniform psychoses)
    Acute deliria and organic psychoses
    Drug-induced psychoses due to hallucinogens and psychostimulants (not
      phencyclidine)
    Nonpsychiatric uses: nausea and vomiting; movement disorders
Possibly effective
    Brief use for episodes of severe dyscontrol or apparent psychosis in some
      personality disorders
Long-term use (> 3 mos)
Effective
    Schizophrenia
    Gilles de la Tourette syndrome
    Treatment-resistant bipolar disorder
    Huntington's disease and other movement disorders
    Chronic organic psychoses
Possibly effective
    Paranoid disorders
    Childhood psychoses

The probable heterogeneity of schizophrenia has made drug studies difficult. Success in one small unidentified subgroup might be masked by failure of the same treatment in a larger group of individuals diagnosed as schizophrenic. Despite these difficulties, multiple clinical studies with antipsychotic drugs have proved that they are helpful for the majority of schizophrenic patients both for acute exacerbations and for long-term maintenance. Rigorous studies of clozapine have shown that it may be of particular benefit in chronic schizophrenia refractory to other antipsychotic drugs; case series and anecdotal reports suggest it may also be effective in refractory atypical psychoses, such as schizoaffective disorder.

Symptoms of schizophrenia are often divided into positive symptoms (i.e., symptoms that are not present in normal human cognitions, perceptions, or affect [e.g., hallucinations, delusions, and thought disorder]) and negative or deficit symptoms (i.e., loss of qualities normally present in healthy individuals [e.g., impoverishment of thought, deficits of attention, blunted affect, and lack of initiative]). It has often been stated that antipsychotic drugs are more effective in treating positive than negative symptoms. However, when examined carefully, this generalization is not entirely accurate; negative symptoms that occur as symptoms of an acute exacerbation of schizophrenia often respond well to antipsychotic drugs. Moreover, many patients continue to have some positive symptoms, such as hallucinations and delusions, despite antipsychotic medication. The expectation that all positive symptoms should respond to antipsychotic therapy has led to the use of excessive doses in some patients. However, it does appear to be true that negative symptoms that characterize the patient's chronic course, that is, negative or deficit symptoms that are present even at times when positive symptoms are minimal, tend to be relatively refractory to antipsychotic drug treatment. Although not all clinicians and studies agree, it appears that clozapine may be more effective than typical antipsychotic drugs in diminishing such negative symptoms. Whether risperidone has special efficacy in treating such negative symptoms remains to be established.

It is also important to recall that side effects of antipsychotic drugs can mimic both positive and negative features of schizophrenia. Akathisia can be indistinguishable from agitation and anxiety (positive symptoms), and the parkinsonian effects of antipsychotics (e.g., bradykinesia, akinesia, masked facies) can masquerade as negative symptoms of the disorder. Indeed the D_2 dopamine receptor antagonism of typical antipsychotic drugs, by causing even subtle akinesia, may create a therapeutic ceiling effect vis-à-vis negative symptoms in some patients.

Acute Exacerbations of Schizophrenia

When a patient with known or suspected schizophrenia develops an exacerbation of psychotic symptoms, it is important to consider all possible causes. These include worsening course of illness (despite medication), noncompliance with medication, a superimposed medical disorder, a superimposed depression, drug abuse, psychosocial crises, or toxic effects of the antipsychotic drugs (especially akathisia or neuroleptic-induced catatonia). If the exacerbation involves florid psychotic symptoms, the treatment is the same as that for acute psychosis (see Therapeutic Usage, p. 22).

Identification, if possible, of the cause for the exacerbation is both helpful in treatment of acute relapse and necessary for long-term planning. If noncompliance is the problem, it is often helpful for the physician to explore with the patient the reasons for avoiding medication. If the physician and patient agree that compliance could be improved with injectable drug preparations, the use of long-acting depot preparations may be indicated. If drug abuse or an intercurrent medical or psychiatric illness (such as depression) is to blame, specific treatment is necessary. Failure to address psychosocial factors in relapse (e.g., family problems or lack of an adequate living situation) will predispose the patient to further difficulties.

Long-Term Treatment of Schizophrenia

Many studies have shown that long-term treatment with antipsychotic drugs increases the time between exacerbations among schizophrenic patients who respond to short-term treatment. The relapse rate for schizophrenic patients who are not on maintenance antipsychotic drugs may be as high as 50% at 6 months and 65–80% at 12 months, whereas for those maintained on antipsychotic drugs, the relapse rate may be 10–15% at 6 months and no higher than 25% at 12 months.

Since long-term treatment with typical antipsychotic drugs brings with it the risk of TD, the clinician should carefully consider the risks and benefits of long-term treatment with each patient. Given its morbidity, however, most patients with well-diagnosed schizophrenia will have net benefit from long-term treatment. Although the literature is not clear, it appears that perhaps 20–40% of patients with schizophrenia respond poorly, if at all, to typical antipsychotic drugs. While such patients may represent one or more subgroups who are pathophysiologically distinct, there is currently no known method of subclassifying such patients. It is important to reassess the diagnosis of refractory patients altogether, considering such possibilities as complex partial seizures, Wilson's disease, and Huntington's disease.

Some refractory patients have received extraordinarily high antipsychotic doses, often more reflective of physician frustration than appropriate therapy. There is no evidence of extra benefit at very high doses of antipsychotic drugs, although side effects are clearly worsened. Currently, for patients who have failed to respond to adequate doses of a typical antipsychotic drug, a trial of clozapine is indicated. As described previously, clozapine is the only antipsychotic drug that has been found to be effective for substantial numbers of patients with schizophrenia who have proved refractory to other antipsychotic drugs.

Manic Episodes

Although lithium may be the best choice for the treatment of mania (see Chap. 4), antipsychotic drugs often play an important role in the acute phase of manic episodes.

Acute Mania

Although mild episodes of mania can usually be treated with lithium or an anticonvulsant alone, such drugs may not be effective for 10–14 days or more. Thus, when mania is accompanied by disruptive or dangerous behavior requiring rapid treatment, antipsychotic drugs may prove useful. Severe manic presentations with marked agitation and florid psychotic symptoms are often optimally treated as an acute psychosis (see Therapeutic Usage, p. 22) with antipsychotic drugs in the dosage range of 8–10 mg/day of haloperidol, or the equivalent, and often the concomitant use of a benzodiazepine such as lorazepam or clonazepam. In the meantime, necessary laboratory tests for lithium therapy can be performed and lithium therapy can be started (usually the next day when the renal function is known). Once the patient is on therapeutic doses of lithium (serum level 1.0–1.2 mEq/L for acute episodes) or an anticonvulsant, and there is marked symptomatic improvement, the antipsychotic drug can be slowly tapered. Should symptoms reemerge during the tapering, the antipsychotic drug can be increased again until the patient has been stable for 1–2 weeks.

Long-Term Treatment of Mania

Because of the success of lithium and the anticonvulsants valproate and carbamazepine for many bipolar patients, long-term use of antipsychotic drugs for prophylaxis of manic-depressive illnesses should be reserved for a small number of refractory patients, weighing short- and long-term toxicity with therapeutic benefit. (There is suggestive but inconclusive evidence that patients with mood disorders may have a greater susceptibility to TD than patients with schizophrenia.) Some bipolar patients may benefit from brief courses of antipsychotic drugs when "breakthrough" symptoms of mania emerge despite lithium prophylaxis. A small number of patients with unremitting or rapidly cycling manic symptoms (despite other treatments) will require maintenance antipsychotic medication. There are now reports and clinical experience to suggest that some such refractory bipolar patients benefit from long-term treatment with clozapine, which appears to carry little or no risk of TD.

Depression with Psychotic Features

Evidence from controlled studies suggests that depression with psychotic features is more effectively treated with the combination of an antidepressant and an antipsychotic drug (70–80% response rate) than with either class of drug alone (30–40% response rate). Electroconvulsive therapy appears to be the most effective treatment and is the treatment of choice if pharmacologic treatment fails or if the severity of symptoms demands extremely rapid treatment. In combined treatment, a high-potency antipsychotic drug is often combined with a tricyclic antidepressant. A high-potency antipsychotic drug should be used to minimize additive anticholinergic toxicity with cyclic antidepressants. Combinations of antipsychotic drugs with selective serotonin reuptake inhibitors (SSRIs) may also prove effective, but there is some concern that SSRIs may be less effective than tricyclic antidepressants for the most severely depressed patients. Depression with psychotic features is more fully discussed in Chapter 3.

Schizoaffective Disorder

As defined in DSM-IV, schizoaffective disorder probably represents a heterogeneous group of patients rather than a single disease entity. The diagnosis is applied to patients who have periods of major manic or depressive symptoms or both, but who have prominent psychotic symptoms even at times when they are relatively free of affective symptoms. Clinically, affective symptoms often respond to lithium, antidepressants, or an anticonvulsant. Psychotic symptoms, especially those that occur between episodes of mood disorder, generally require treatment with antipsychotic medication. The dosages of antipsychotic medication for both acute florid symptoms and chronic maintenance are the same as for the analogous stages of schizophrenia. Preliminary reports suggest that clozapine may be effective for schizoaffective patients. Use of lithium in this disorder is discussed in Chapter 4, anticonvulsants in Chapter 5.

Schizophreniform Disorder

As defined by the DSM-IV, schizophreniform disorder involves overt psychotic symptoms of less than 6 months' duration, with return to the premorbid level of functioning. The onset of symptoms tends to be rapid, rather than insidious, and patients may demonstrate confusion or perplexity at the height of their syndrome. Many, but not all, such patients lack the flat affect of typical schizophrenia.

Schizophreniform patients represent a heterogeneous group. Depending on the precise population studied, some investigators find them to represent largely patients with atypical mood disorders; others find them to be more heterogeneous, with perhaps half manifesting schizophrenia over time. The early stages of treatment for schizophreniform disorder are the same as for any acute psychosis (see Therapeutic Usage, p. 22). Given that the long-term prognosis for recovery of many of these patients is good, an attempt should be made to taper and discontinue antipsychotic drugs entirely if symptoms fully remit. Many patients who meet criteria for schizophreniform disorder will benefit from lithium or anticonvulsants, both acutely and long-term (see Chaps. 4 and 5).

Delusional (Paranoid) Disorders

Patients with delusional (paranoid) disorder are often difficult to treat. They generally deny that they have a mental disorder, and their pervasive suspiciousness often extends to physicians and medical treatment. As a result, they are frequently brought to treatment by someone else and are often noncompliant. It may improve compliance if medication is offered as a way of helping patients cope with anxiety and stress or other complaints they might have rather than confronting them about their delusions, at least at the initiation of treatment.

Antipsychotic drugs are effective in some patients with delusional disorder, especially in those whose symptoms are of recent onset. For patients with chronic, systematized delusions, the response rate may be lower than for those with a more recent onset. Low doses of antipsychotic drugs should be used initially (e.g., haloperidol, 5 mg/day or the equivalent) to minimize side effects and enhance compliance. Doses greater than the equivalent of haloperidol 10 mg/day do not appear to be warranted. If the only benefit after a 6- to 8-week trial of adequate doses of an antipsychotic drug is anxiolysis, serious consideration should be given to discontinuing the medication because of the risk of TD. In such patients, benzodiazepines may be useful because of their anxiolytic and sedative properties, without the short- and long-term neurologic toxicity inherent in the antipsychotics. Consideration should be given to a trial of antidepressants or lithium if affective symptomatology is apparent or if there is a clear family history of mood disorder.

Delirium and Acute Organic Psychoses

Delirium, acute confusional states, and toxic/metabolic encephalopathy are among the many terms that have been used to describe a clinical syndrome that consists of acute global depression of cerebral function generally accompanied by abnormalities in arousal. Delirium may result from a wide variety of medical causes, many of which are medical emergencies. The cornerstone of treatment for delirium is supportive care while specific therapy for the underlying disorder is provided. Because delirious patients are unpredictable and may either harm themselves by falling or by pulling out necessary lines and tubes in a hospital setting, or harm others by striking out, restraints are generally indicated. Pending the results of specific therapy for an underlying disorder or while waiting for an offending drug to be metabolized and excreted, symptomatic use of sedatives may be necessary, although their use should be minimized if possible, especially when the diagnosis is unclear. The choice of sedative will be dictated by the cause of the delirium and the patient's medical status.

Delirium due to ethanol, benzodiazepine, or barbiturate withdrawal is best treated with a cross-reactive agent, generally a benzodiazepine (see Chap. 6). Antipsychotic drugs are not effective treatments for ethanol withdrawal. When delirium is caused by anticholinergic drugs, it is also wise to avoid antipsychotics because of the risk of increasing anticholinergic toxicity. For many other causes of delirium, especially in medically fragile patients, haloperidol is often the agent of choice because it has little effect on the cardiovascular system, little effect on respiratory drive, and very low anticholinergic potency. Low-potency antipsychotic drugs lower the seizure threshold, increase the risk of postural hypotension, and may be strongly anticholinergic; thus they should be avoided. In older patients, doses of haloperidol as low as 0.5 mg bid may be effective in symptomatic treatment of delirium. In younger patients, much higher doses may be required at least initially (doses of 2–5 mg may be given parenterally q30–60min as needed). The major liability of haloperidol, especially in the elderly, is the emergence of parkinsonian symptoms. When elderly patients are given antipsychotics, they should be monitored frequently for cogwheel rigidity, changes in gait, and the development of masked facies. Late reemergence of agitation while a patient is on haloperidol should raise the suspicion of akathisia.

Dementia

In treating patients with dementing illnesses, antipsychotic drugs have two major roles: treating complicating psychotic symptoms that may occur (e.g., paranoid delusions) and treating severe agitation that cannot be helped by manipulation of the patient's environment. Low doses of a high-potency antipsychotic drug such as haloperidol or fluphenazine (0.5–2.0 mg/day) are often effective.

Psychotic Symptoms with Parkinson's Disease

Patients with idiopathic Parkinson's disease may develop psychotic symptoms, associated with L-dopa therapy or in the context of dementia. Low doses of thioridazine (e.g., 10–25 mg/day) have been used in the past, with careful monitoring for postural hypotension, anticholinergic symptoms, or worsening of the movement disorder. Several case series and clinical experience suggest that clozapine may be the most effective treatment for psychosis in Parkinson's disease if the patient can tolerate the side effects (including anticholinergic effects) and if weekly blood drawing can be arranged.

Gilles de la Tourette Syndrome

Gilles de la Tourette syndrome is characterized by multiple motor and phonic tics, which develop during childhood and are chronic in duration. The nature and severity of the symptoms vary markedly over time and among individuals. In addition to motor and phonic symptoms, patients may have difficulty with concentration, impulsiveness, obsessions, and compulsions.

When severe, this disorder is disabling and may require long-term drug treatment. Both haloperidol and pimozide have been used in the treatment of Gilles de la Tourette syndrome. Because of pimozide's cardiac side effects (increased QTc interval with risk of torsades de pointes ventricular tachycardia), the FDA has limited its dosage approval to 0.3 mg/kg or 20 mg/day, whichever is less. At these doses, serious cardiac side effects are rare. A well-designed placebo-controlled crossover study (Shapiro et al., 1989) confirmed that both haloperidol and pimozide are effective for Gilles de la Tourette syndrome at a mean dose of approximately 4 mg of haloperidol and 11 mg of pimozide. In the crossover portion of the study, haloperidol appeared to be slightly more effective than pimozide, without significantly worse side effects. Based on prior studies, however, it cannot be stated with certainty that haloperidol has advantages over pimozide; thus, the clinician should use the drug that is best tolerated by the patient. Haloperidol is usually begun at 1 mg/day in a single nightly dose, with slow dosage increases (e.g., 1 or 2 mg/wk) until adequate symptom control is attained. Dosages above 10 mg/day of haloperidol are rarely warranted. Because of the risk of cardiac toxicity, patients who are not optimally treated with 20 mg/day of pimozide should probably be switched to haloperidol. Long-term treatment studies with both of these agents are much needed. For patients who cannot tolerate antipsychotic drugs, clonidine may prove to be a useful alternative (see Chap. 7).

Personality Disorders

Given their lack of proven effectiveness in treating personality disorders and the risk of TD, the antipsychotic drugs should be prescribed only when other treatments (including nonpharmacologic therapies) have failed. The clinician should choose observable target symptoms that may be responsive to antipsychotic drugs. These symptoms should be monitored carefully, and the drug discontinued if there is no clear improvement. In particular, the antipsychotic drugs have been used in personality disorder patients during periods of apparent psychosis and in treating episodes of accelerated impulsiveness, rage, and assaultiveness. When psychotic symptoms emerge, it is important to reconsider the diagnosis. Consider the possibility of a mood disorder, complex partial seizures, drug abuse, or factitious symptoms; therapies other than antipsychotic medications would be preferable in such situations. When antipsychotic drugs are used, the duration of treatment should be brief. There are no established guidelines, but dosages greater than the equivalent of

10 mg/day of haloperidol do not appear to be warranted. The possible use of carbamazepine for episodes of dyscontrol in personality-disorder patients is currently a matter of study (see Chap. 5).

THERAPEUTIC USAGE

Choosing an Antipsychotic Drug

All of the compounds approved as antipsychotic drugs in the United States are effective. Except for clozapine, which appears to be more effective than the others in the treatment of schizophrenia, the antipsychotic drugs differ only in their potency (the dosage needed to produce the desired effect) and side effects. Antipsychotic drugs that are most potent tend to produce more extrapyramidal effects (the high-potency drug risperidone appears to be an exception), and those that are less potent produce more sedation, postural hypotension, and anticholinergic effects (see Table 2-1). For example, 8 mg of haloperidol and 400 mg of chlorpromazine are equivalent with regard to antipsychotic efficacy; however, the patient receiving haloperidol would be more likely to develop extrapyramidal symptoms, and the patient on chlorpromazine would be more likely to feel sedated and to develop postural hypotension.

Since, with the exception of clozapine, there is no difference in the therapeutic effectiveness of these drugs, their side effect profiles should be a central consideration when starting a patient on antipsychotic treatment. (Most physicians will not use all antipsychotic drugs routinely in practice. At the minimum, a general physician should master the use of one standard high-potency drug, such as haloperidol, and one low-potency drug, such as thioridazine; at the minimum, a psychiatrist should, in addition, master the use of clozapine and risperidone.)

A patient who has responded well to a particular antipsychotic drug in the past is likely to do well on the same drug again. On the other hand, if a patient has a history of severe EPS or other troublesome side effects with a particular drug, it would be best to try another compound with a different side effect profile. Some patients may benefit from the sedation provided by chlorpromazine or thioridazine (e.g., the young manic patient with severe insomnia), but it is generally preferable to use a less sedating compound combined with temporary use of a benzodiazepine (e.g., clonazepam) to achieve sedation, so that when the acute episode passes, the patient is not saddled with unwanted side effects.

For certain groups of patients (Table 2-4), side effects can aid in the selection of a drug. Severely suicidal patients should not be given thioridazine, mesoridazine, or pimozide, since these are the antipsychotics that can be cardiotoxic in overdose. Patients with glaucoma, prostatism, or other contraindications to anticholinergic drugs should not be given low-potency drugs, especially thioridazine, nor should low-potency drugs be given to patients taking other anticholinergic compounds such as tricyclic antidepressants. Clozapine can only be administered to patients who are adequately compliant so that they will submit to weekly blood drawing.

Use of Antipsychotic Drugs

Since antipsychotic drugs can produce striking changes in the thinking, language, and behavior (including motor behavior) of the

Table 2-4. Recommended agents for certain patient groups

Condition	Recommendation
Cardiac illness	Avoid low-potency agents and pimozide
Elderly	Use low dosages of high-potency agents; caution with risperidone due to hypotension
Refractory drug-induced EPS	Consider risperidone, thioridazine, clozapine
Parkinson's disease	Thioridazine if tolerated; consider clozapine
Suicidal patients	Avoid thioridazine, mesoridazine, or pimozide
Delirium	Avoid anticholinergic drugs (especially thioridazine)
History of dystonia	Use thioridazine or high-potency drug plus anticholinergic
Refractory schizophrenia	Clozapine

patients who receive them, it is critical that a thorough physical and mental status examination be performed before initiating therapy. In many psychotic disorders, the mental status may fluctuate markedly; thus a period of drug-free observation may be helpful when the diagnosis is unclear. A reliable history must always supplement the mental status examination. In all cases, but especially when the diagnosis is unclear, it is important to note objectively rateable target symptoms that can be monitored throughout treatment with antipsychotic drugs. The physician must have a clear notion of the symptoms that are likely to respond specifically to antipsychotic drugs and the symptoms (e.g., anxiety) that may be better treated by other classes of drugs.

The latency of response of psychotic symptoms such as delusions, hallucinations, and bizarre behavior is usually greater than 5 days, with nonspecific tranquilization and sedation occurring more rapidly. Full benefit in antipsychotic-responsive disorders usually takes at least 2–6 weeks. Unfortunately, physicians are often impatient in treating psychoses because the patients tend to be disruptive. Thus, premature dosage increases often occur, and when symptoms finally remit, the time course of improvement is often mistaken for a "requirement" for high doses of antipsychotic drugs. Thus if dangerous behavior must be rapidly controlled, the physician may choose to increase the antipsychotic drug dosage temporarily to exploit its nonspecific sedative and tranquilizing properties or perhaps more wisely choose to use an adjunctive benzodiazepine as needed. In either case, once the acute symptoms subside, the extra sedating dosages should be tapered and an optimal antipsychotic drug dosage established.

Specific Clinical Situations

In the treatment of any psychotic disorder, certain paradigmatic situations arise, each requiring a distinct approach to the use of antipsychotic drugs. These include (1) acute psychoses in which the symptoms may constitute a medical emergency, (2) long-term treatment aimed at minimizing residual symptoms or prophylaxis of recurrent psychosis, and (3) use of antipsychotics on an "as needed" (prn) basis.

Acute Psychosis

Acute psychosis is a clinical syndrome that may be caused by a wide variety of disorders (Table 2-5). Typically, patients present with rapid onset (days to weeks) of psychotic symptoms (e.g., hallucinations, delusions, ideas of reference), agitation, insomnia, and often

Table 2-5.   Causes of acute psychotic syndromes

Major psychiatric disorders
    Acute exacerbation of schizophrenia
    Atypical psychoses (e.g., schizophreniform)
    Depression with psychotic features
    Mania

Drug abuse and withdrawal
    Alcohol withdrawal
    Amphetamines and cocaine
    Phencyclidine (PCP) and hallucinogens
    Sedative-hypnotic withdrawal

Prescription drugs
    Anticholinergic agents
    Digitalis toxicity
    Glucocorticoids and adrenocorticotropic hormone (ACTH)
    Isoniazid
    L-Dopa and other dopamine agonists
    Nonsteroidal anti-inflammatory agents
    Withdrawal from MAOIs

Other toxic agents
    Carbon disulfide
    Heavy metals

Neurologic causes
    AIDS encephalopathy
    Brain tumor
    Complex partial seizures
    Early Alzheimer's or Pick's disease
    Huntington's disease
    Hypoxic encephalopathy
    Infectious viral encephalitis
    Lupus cerebritis
    Neurosyphilis
    Stroke
    Wilson's disease

Metabolic causes
    Acute intermittent porphyria
    Cushing's syndrome
    Early hepatic encephalopathy
    Hypo- and hypercalcemia
    Hypoglycemia
    Hypo- and hyperthyroidism
    Paraneoplastic syndromes (limbic encephalitis)

Nutritional causes
    Niacin deficiency (pellagra)
    Thiamine deficiency (Wernicke-Korsakoff syndrome)
    Vitamin B_{12} deficiency

hostility and/or combativeness. It is important to rule out acute medical illness by obtaining as much history as possible, monitoring vital signs, performing a physical examination, and ordering necessary laboratory work.

During an acute presentation (having excluded a medical disorder), it may still be difficult to make a definitive psychiatric diagnosis. Because a diagnosis cannot be made from mental status alone, and acutely psychotic patients often are poor historians, a definitive diagnosis may be difficult to establish immediately. To make a diagnosis, the following factors need to be considered:

1. Clinical presentation
2. Medical history, including any prescription or other drug use
3. Physical examination and any relevant laboratory tests
4. Past psychiatric history
5. Mental status examination
6. Baseline of premorbid functioning
7. Time course of onset of symptoms and overall duration of illness
8. History of prior treatment response, especially to antidepressants, lithium, or electroconvulsive therapy
9. Family history of psychiatric or neurologic disorders

When patients are extremely agitated, combative, or hyperactive, it may be necessary to begin treatment before a definitive diagnosis can be made. Fortunately, most acute primary psychotic disorders, and many psychoses secondary to medical and neurologic disorders, respond to antipsychotic drug treatment regardless of the specific disorder. Optimal long-term treatment requires that a correct diagnosis be made. In addition, it is important to identify conditions that might be worsened by some or all of the antipsychotic agents (e.g., low-potency antipsychotic drugs may worsen symptoms of phencyclidine toxicity or anticholinergic delirium; catatonic states may be caused by neuroleptic toxicity in some patients).

Since acutely psychotic patients are potentially dangerous to themselves and others, even if not immediately agitated or threatening, rapid treatment is an important goal. In the 1970s and 1980s, many clinicians utilized very high-dose antipsychotic drug regimens (rapid neuroleptization) on the assumption that such doses would provide more rapid control of major psychotic symptoms than "standard doses." This impression was *not* borne out when carefully scrutinized. In fact, since high-dose regimens produced more side effects, they often clouded the diagnostic picture in short-term treatment (e.g., by producing catatoniclike states or akathisia) and compromised patient acceptance of therapy in long-term treatment. In addition, there is a poorly substantiated impression that high-dose, high-potency neuroleptic regimens might increase the risk of neuroleptic malignant syndrome.

For the clinician, the question is: What dose of antipsychotic should be used? Unfortunately, the dose-response relationship for antipsychotic therapy has been difficult to establish with certainty either in good-prognosis psychoses, such as mania, or in poorer-prognosis psychoses, such as florid presentations of schizophrenia, because the clinical and ethical need to gain rapid control over the symptoms oftens precludes controlled studies. Studies of acute mania suggest that the vast majority of patients improve on doses equivalent to less than 10 mg/day of haloperidol. Since the occurrence and severity of EPS are dose-related, it is reasonable not to exceed the equivalent of 8–10 mg/day of haloperidol in the short-term treatment of acute mania. (Therapy with lithium and/or an anticonvulsant would likely be instituted concomitantly.) Optimal dosage in schizophrenia and schizoaffective disorder has been addressed in several recent studies. In one study (Van Putten et al., 1990), patients were treated with fixed doses of haloperidol (5, 10, or 20 mg/day) for 4 weeks. The 20-mg dose was superior to the 5-mg dose throughout the trial and was marginally superior to the 10-mg dose after the first 2 weeks of treatment. By the second week, however, the group given 20 mg/day experienced symptomatic worsening with respect to blunted affect, motor retardation, and emotional withdrawal. In addition, a significantly higher percentage of patients on the 20-mg dose left the hospital against medical advice than those on lower doses. Although the study was flawed because the staff was not blind to the dosage, it suggests that at high doses, toxicity of antipsychotics may outweigh benefits.

Based on available studies and clinical experience, recommendations for the clinical management of acute psychoses can be made. The dose of a standard antipsychotic drug that can be administered is limited by side effects that may have adverse consequences on the overall course. Doses of 8–10 mg/day of haloperidol or the equivalent are likely to be effective for mania and other good-prognosis psychoses. For schizophrenia and schizoaffective disorder, doses of 10–15 mg/day of haloperidol or the equivalent appear to be optimal in nonrefractory patients, beginning with the lower dose. Risperidone 6 mg/day is an alternative.

If a high-potency antipsychotic drug is used, an anticholinergic drug should be added as prophylaxis against dystonia; benztropine mesylate, 2 mg bid, may be used. Evidence from various studies has demonstrated that such a regimen decreases the incidence of acute dystonia, which is a problem particularly in individuals younger than 40. If anticholinergic side effects become a problem, the dosage can be decreased to benztropine, 1 mg bid.

It should be recognized that a substantial number of patients with schizophrenia do not benefit from standard antipsychotic drugs. For these patients, very high doses are likely to produce more serious side effects with no therapeutic benefit. Schizophrenic patients who have been unresponsive to two standard antipsychotic drugs deserve a trial of clozapine. Approaches to refractory mania are discussed in Chapters 4 and 5.

Even for responsive patients, a clinical problem remains. At the recommended doses of antipsychotic drugs, many patients will remain agitated in the short term and may exhibit potentially dangerous behaviors. Therefore in acute psychoses, in addition to effective doses of an antipsychotic drug, short-term use of sedatives may be required.

For example, a patient might initially be given 5 mg of haloperidol IM or as the liquid concentrate (to ensure adequate absorption) as part of a 5-mg bid regimen. If the patient continues to be agitated, an adjunctive benzodiazepine would provide safe and reliable sedation. Lorazepam, which has a relatively short half-life, has no active metabolites, and is well absorbed intramuscularly, is a good choice. Other clinicians prefer the longer-acting benzodiazepine clonazepam, which has the disadvantage of lacking a parenteral form. Lorazepam, 1–2 mg PO or IM, or clonazepam, 0.5–1.0 mg PO, could be given every 2 hours as needed to quiet an agitated patient. A rare patient may require higher dosages of sedatives. Benzodiazepines appear to be relatively free of dangerous side effects if used carefully in the short term. The physician should monitor carefully the course of psychotic symptoms over the first 2 weeks of treatment, being alert to the fact that as the acute psychosis improves, the requirement of adjunctive benzodiazepine is likely to decrease. It is recommended that the sedative drug be tapered as agitation subsides.

Long-Term Use

Because many patients for whom antipsychotic drugs are effective have chronic or relapsing illnesses, long-term use of these drugs may be indicated. Because with typical antipsychotic drugs the danger of producing TD is significant, the clinician should continually monitor the duration of treatment and consider alternative treatments whenever possible.

It is difficult to recommend maintenance dosages based on the literature because of the extreme variability of the studies. One comprehensive review (Baldessarini and Davis, 1980) found no correlation between dosage and effectiveness for long-term therapy, suggesting that even the lowest dosages reported (about 125 mg/day of chlorpromazine) exceeded the minimum effective dosage and that higher dosages offered no further benefit.

For oral medication, it is likely that dosages in the range of 2–4 mg/day of haloperidol or the equivalent are more than adequate for most patients. Throughout the course of long-term treatment, it is best to reconsider the dosage, always striving for the lowest effective dosage. This strategy is preferable to the use of "drug holidays," which are of no proven benefit and may increase the risk of TD.

LONG-ACTING PREPARATIONS.   When patients with schizophrenia or other chronic psychoses relapse because of noncompliance, consideration should be given to the use of long-acting antipsychotic preparations. Of course, in some patients, noncompliance may respond to psychosocial measures, obviating the need for depot antipsychotic drugs.

The depot preparations available in the United States are fluphenazine decanoate and haloperidol decanoate. Controlled studies of fluphenazine decanoate have covered a 100-fold range in dosage (1.25–125 mg q2wk). High doses (> 25 mg q2wk) appear to be associated with an inferior outcome. Although these studies may have been skewed by assignment of sicker patients to higher dosages, the general impression is that the dosages used in current clinical practice are often too high.

There are no ideal conversion ratios from oral dosages to depot preparations of fluphenazine. One reasonable estimate is that 0.5 ml of fluphenazine decanoate given every two weeks is equivalent to 10.0 mg/day of fluphenazine hydrochloride. For haloperidol decanoate, the ratio of decanoate to oral dose is about 10–15 : 1, so that 150 mg of the decanoate given every four weeks is equivalent to 10 mg/day of oral haloperidol. Since these conversions are only approximate, individual dosage adjustments will have to be made.

Because these are long-acting preparations, patients should be exposed to the oral form of the drug prior to their first injection to minimize the possibility of a long-lasting idiosyncratic reaction. It is safest to start long-acting agents at low dosages and then carefully adjust them to maximize the safety of therapy and minimize side effects. Since fluphenazine and haloperidol are high-potency antipsychotic drugs, extrapyramidal side effects are to be expected. Safe and effective use of these compounds can be achieved using the following recommendations:

1. Ensure that the patient has had a test of the drug orally to make certain that it is tolerated.
2. Start injections at low doses, for example, 5.0–12.5 mg (0.2–0.5 ml) of fluphenazine decanoate or 50–100 mg (1–2 ml) of haloperidol decanoate. Give fluphenazine decanoate q2wk and haloperidol decanoate q4wk.
3. With the initial low doses, oral supplementation may temporarily be necessary. Do not increase doses of the depot preparation too rapidly because steady state is only reached after 4–5 dosing intervals.
4. Average effective dosages are in the range of 12.5 mg (0.5 ml) q2wk for fluphenazine and 150 mg (3 ml) q4wk for haloperidol decanoate.
5. Observe patients for akinesia, "depressionlike" symptoms, or increasing withdrawal. Because these symptoms may be drug-induced, it may be necessary to lower the dosage. Parkinsonism and akathisia are also common and require treatment.
6. Recall that worsening of psychotic symptoms with dosage reduction may not become evident for several weeks; hence, the clinician must monitor patients for an extended period of time before assuming that the reduction has been successful.

PRN Use

Antipsychotic drugs are commonly used on a prn basis for the presence of overt psychotic symptoms or agitation. Although a common practice, using antipsychotics on a prn basis may be irrational. The time course of improvement for psychotic disorders in response to antipsychotic drugs is such that intermittent dosing is unlikely to help and may confuse the physician as to the amount of antipsychotic drug the patient is receiving daily. Patients receiving only intermittent antipsychotic drug doses for psychotic symptoms are likely to do poorly; this would be much like using an SSRI or tricyclic antidepressant on a prn basis.

Frequent examinations by a physician are preferable to long-standing prn orders for antipsychotic drugs that may mask or exacerbate side effects or undiagnosed medical illness. All too often, for example, patients with akathisia are given extra (prn) doses of an antipsychotic drug because their symptoms are misinterpreted by nursing staff as "agitation." If prn medication is needed to provide sedation for an acutely disturbed patient, benzodiazepines (e.g., lorazepam) are generally preferable to prn use of antipsychotic drugs because they are reliably sedating with fewer side effects (see Chap. 6). It should be recalled that even hallucinations may worsen with anxiety, fear, and agitation and are likely to respond to adequate sedation without additional antipsychotic drugs.

Clozapine

In both well-designed clinical trials and clinical experience, clozapine has proved to be effective even for some patients with schizophrenia who do not respond to other antipsychotic drugs. Clozapine has the additional significant advantage of being almost free of EPS and of not causing TD. Thus it has not only produced improvement in previously refractory patients but has also been used effectively in some patients with severe EPS, including akathisia, who could not tolerate typical antipsychotic drugs. In addition to its efficacy for its FDA-approved indication, the treatment of refractory schizophrenia, early reports suggest that it may also have utility in the treatment of refractory schizoaffective disorder, other atypical psychoses, and bipolar disorder. Clozapine has also found use in the treatment of L-dopa–induced psychotic symptoms in patients with Parkinson's disease. It has also been reported that clozapine may improve existing TD, but further data are needed to support this contention.

Unfortunately, clozapine has a rather severe side effect profile in its own right, which limits its general utility. Clozapine was first tested in the 1960s but was withdrawn from general use because of its association with high rates of agranulocytosis. It was initially introduced in the United States in 1990, bundled by its manufacturer with a mandatory program of weekly blood counts. While the programs available for blood count determinations have since been broadened, weekly determination of granulocyte counts is absolutely necessary with clozapine. The rate of agranulocytosis with clozapine has been approximately 1%. Despite appropriate monitoring, there had been seven fatalities due to agranulocytosis in the United States by 1993. More than 95% of cases of agranulocytosis occur within the first 6 months of treatment, with the period of highest risk between weeks 4 and 18. The risk also appears to increase with age and may be higher in women. The mechanism of agranulocytosis is not known.

As previously described, clozapine has a relatively low affinity for D_2 dopamine receptors compared with typical antipsychotic drugs and a higher ratio of affinity for D_4 versus D_2 dopamine receptors than any other antipsychotic drug. Its relatively low affinity for D_2 dopamine receptors is likely responsible for its relative lack of EPS, although its high-affinity antagonism of $5\text{-}HT_2$ serotonin receptors may also play a role. It interacts also with D_1 and D_3 dopamine receptors, alpha$_1$-adrenergic receptors, and muscarinic cholinergic receptors. The mechanism of its unique efficacy remains unknown.

To minimize side effects, clozapine is begun with a single 12.5- or 25-mg daily dose, increased to 25 mg bid, and then increased by no more than 25 mg/day to a dosage of 300–450 mg/day over a period of 2–3 weeks. Dosage should subsequently be increased no more rapidly than weekly in increments no greater than 100 mg. Careful monitoring for significant tachycardia and postural hypotension is important in the first month of treatment. Should these occur, the dosage may be temporarily decreased and then increased again more slowly. Most clozapine-responsive patients are effectively treated at dosages between 300 and 600 mg/day in divided doses. Some patients have been treated with dosages as high as 900 mg/day in divided doses, but at doses of 600 mg and above, the risk of seizures increases significantly (from 1–2% to 3–5%). The optimal duration of a trial to identify clozapine-responsive patients remains unknown. Patients should be treated for at least 12 weeks, and some clinicians would recommend considerably longer (e.g., 6 month) trials of clozapine before declaring the treatment ineffective.

In addition to agranulocytosis, seizures, and postural hypotension, other problematic side effects include sedation, hypersalivation (which may be marked), tachycardia (which may be persistent), constipation, transient hyperthermia, and, similar to most other antipsychotic drugs, weight gain. Eosinophilia without serious consequences has also rarely been reported.

Some patients being discontinued from clozapine to start another antipsychotic drug, such as risperidone, have experienced marked agitation and even rebound psychotic symptoms. The mechanism is unknown but likely represents some type of withdrawal syndrome. Slow tapering of clozapine rather than abrupt termination is recommended, even when switching to another antipsychotic drug.

Plasma concentrations of clozapine may be increased by drugs that inhibit P450 hepatic enzymes, such as cimetidine and SSRIs.

Risperidone

Risperidone, which was recently introduced into the United States, combines high affinity for D_2 dopamine receptors with high affinity for $5-HT_2$ receptors. The high D_2 affinity is similar to haloperidol (rather than clozapine), while the high $5-HT_2$ affinity is similar to clozapine. Risperidone also has high affinity for alpha$_1$-adrenergic receptors, resulting in the tendency to cause postural hypotension, but low affinity for muscarinic cholinergic receptors, making it devoid of anticholinergic effects. If $5-HT_2$ receptor antagonism were the key component to the unique efficacy of clozapine, risperidone might have similar benefits to clozapine with a more benign side effect profile. Based on the studies to date and early clinical experience, however, it appears that while risperidone is an effective antipsychotic medication, it does not have the unique properties of clozapine (i.e., enhanced efficacy and lack of EPS). On the other hand, in early experience, effective doses of risperidone appear to have less tendency to cause EPS than does haloperidol, which would provide a real advantage. Convincing data that risperidone has greater effectiveness for negative symptoms of schizophrenia than standard antipsychotic drugs are not yet available.

Patients are started on 1 mg bid (0.5 mg bid for the elderly or for those with impaired hepatic function). The dosage is increased to 2 mg bid on day two and then 3 mg bid on day three if tolerated by the patient. Dosage increases should be slower in the elderly and in those who experience postural hypotension with initial dosing. Optimal antipsychotic effects for most schizophrenic patients are seen at 6 mg/day in divided doses. If no response is observed after 2–3 weeks, weekly dosage adjustments may be made in increments of 1 mg bid. However, dosages above 10 mg/day do not appear to have any added benefit. The incidence of EPS appears to be dose-related; at dosages of 8 mg/day or greater the incidence of EPS is similar to that of haloperidol.

In addition to postural hypotension, risperidone may produce sedation, asthenia, and difficulty concentrating. Dizziness, galactorrhea, and weight gain have also been reported. As noted, at dosages of 6 mg/day, risperidone appears to cause less EPS than 10 mg/day of haloperidol. Like all D_2 receptor antagonists, risperidone may have the potential to cause TD and neuroleptic malignant syndrome, although it is too early to judge these risks clinically. Risperidone and its metabolite, 9-hydroxyrisperidone, may increase the cardiac QT interval; the clinical significance of this is currently unknown.

USE OF ANTIPSYCHOTIC
DRUGS IN PREGNANCY AND NURSING

Antipsychotic medications achieve significant levels in the fetus and amniotic fluid. The effects of chlorpromazine have been the most carefully studied in pregnancy, although other agents have also been investigated with regard to teratogenicity. No clear patterns of toxicity or teratogenicity have emerged. Given the relative paucity of safety data, it is best if antipsychotic agents can be avoided in pregnancy, especially in the first trimester. Nonetheless, there are situations in which failure to treat the mother creates a graver risk to the fetus than the established risk of antipsychotic drugs. Careful clinical judgment is required.

There are well-documented problems with the use of antipsychotics in late pregnancy. Chlorpromazine has been associated with an increased risk of neonatal jaundice. In addition, there are reports that mothers treated with antipsychotic drugs have given birth to infants with EPS. The washout time for these drugs in the fetus is at least 7–10 days. Therefore, to avoid EPS in the newborn, it has been recommended that the antipsychotic be discontinued 2 weeks before the due date. If the discontinuance predisposes the expectant mother to severe psychotic symptoms, the clinician must carefully weigh the risks of the psychotic disorder against the potential for neuroleptic toxicity in the child.

Antipsychotics are secreted in breast milk. A nursing infant of a mother treated with antipsychotics is therefore at risk for the development of EPS. Since the effect of antipsychotic drugs on development is unknown, mothers who must take antipsychotic agents should be discouraged from breast-feeding.

USE IN THE ELDERLY

The elderly have slower hepatic metabolism of antipsychotic drugs (pharmacokinetic changes) and increased sensitivity of the brain to dopamine antagonism and anticholinergic effects (pharmacodynamic changes). Thus, lower dosages should be used, and longer waiting periods should be respected before increasing doses. High-potency antipsychotic drugs are less likely than low-potency drugs to cause anticholinergic symptoms such as constipation, urinary retention, tachycardia, sedation, and confusion or to cause postural hypotension. Unfortunately, high-potency antipsychotic drugs have a high likelihood of causing drug-induced parkinsonism in the elderly. Low dosages should therefore be the rule; dosages in the range of 0.5–2.0 mg/day of haloperidol are often adequate in the elderly.

SIDE EFFECTS AND TOXICITY

Although the antipsychotic drugs have a high therapeutic index (they are much safer in terms of lethality than lithium, the tricyclic antidepressants, or monoamine oxidase inhibitors), they have many serious side effects that complicate therapy.

Neurologic Side Effects

Acute Dystonia

CLINICAL PRESENTATION. Acute dystonia is most likely to occur within the first week of treatment. There is a higher incidence in

Table 2-6.   Commonly used antiparkinsonian drugs

Drug	Usual dosage range
Anticholinergic drugs	
Benztropine (Cogentin)	1–2 mg bid
Biperiden (Akineton)	1–3 mg bid
Trihexyphenidyl (Artane, Tremin)	1–3 mg tid
Anticholinergic antihistamine	
Diphenhydramine (Benadryl)	25 mg bid–qid
	50 mg bid
Dopamine-releasing agent	
Amantadine (Symmetrel)	100 mg bid–tid

patients under 40, in males, and in patients on high-potency antipsychotic drugs. Patients may develop acute muscular rigidity and cramping, usually in the musculature of the neck, tongue, face, and back. Occasionally, patients report the subacute onset (3–6 hours) of tongue "thickness" or difficulty in swallowing. Opisthotonos and oculogyric crises may also occur. Acute dystonia can be very uncomfortable, frightening to patients, and occasionally it has serious sequelae; muscular cramps can be severe enough to cause joint dislocation, and most dangerously, laryngeal dystonia can occur with compromise of the airway. Like other EPS, acute dystonia is unlikely with clozapine.

TREATMENT. Anticholinergic drugs (Table 2-6), such as benztropine, 2 mg IM or IV, or diphenhydramine, 50 mg IM or IV, usually bring rapid relief. Benztropine is preferred because it lacks the antihistaminic effects of diphenhydramine. If there is no effect in 20 minutes, a repeat injection is indicated. If the dystonia is still unresponsive after two injections, a benzodiazepine, such as lorazepam 1 mg IM or IV, may be tried. In cases of laryngeal dystonia with airway compromise, repeat dosing should occur at shorter intervals unless the dystonia resolves. The patient should receive 4 mg of benztropine IV within 10 minutes and then 1–2 mg of lorazepam slowly IV if needed.

With reversal of dystonia, antipsychotic medication can be continued, but standing doses of an anticholinergic drug (e.g., benztropine, 2 mg bid) should be prescribed for 2 weeks (see Table 2-6). If a second dystonic reaction occurs despite the use of an anticholinergic, the clinician may opt to change to a low-potency antipsychotic (e.g., thioridazine). There is evidence that the prophylactic use of benztropine, 2 mg bid, begun at the same time as the antipsychotic drug, significantly reduces the incidence of dystonia. Recent literature describes the abuse potential of anticholinergic drugs. The clinician should be aware of this in prescribing anticholinergics to patients who have a history of substance abuse.

Antipsychotic Drug-Induced Parkinsonism

CLINICAL PRESENTATION. Symptoms include bradykinesia, rigidity, cogwheeling, tremor, masked facies, stooped posture, festinating gait, and drooling. Onset is usually after several weeks of therapy and is more common in the elderly and with high-potency drugs, with the exception of risperidone. When these side effects are severe, akinesia, which can be indistinguishable from catatonia, may develop. Parkinsonian effects are very rare with clozapine.

TREATMENT. A fixed dose of antiparkinsonian drug should be prescribed, and the antipsychotic drug dosage should be decreased to the lowest that is effective for the patient. In elderly patients, lower doses of antiparkinsonians should be used (e.g., benztropine, 1 mg bid). A switch to a low-potency antipsychotic (especially thioridazine) may help in some cases. Since there is some evidence that long-term use of anticholinergics may increase the risk of TD, periodic attempts should be made to wean these drugs in patients on maintenance therapy. When parkinsonian effects become very severe (e.g., akinesia), the antipsychotic should be discontinued until the side effect resolves and then resumed at lower doses if necessary.

Akathisia

CLINICAL PRESENTATION. Akathisia is experienced subjectively as an intensely unpleasant need to move. Patients often appear restless with symptoms of anxiety, agitation, or both. It can be very difficult to distinguish akathisia from anxiety related to the psychotic disorder. Increased restlessness following the institution of antipsychotics should always raise the question of akathisia. Recent evidence suggests that akathisia may be more prevalent in patients treated with antipsychotic drugs than previously thought. Akathisia is a leading cause of noncompliance and treatment refusal. As with parkinsonism, akathisia is only very rarely seen with clozapine.

TREATMENT. Antipsychotic drugs should be decreased to the minimum effective dose. Low-potency antipsychotics, especially thioridazine, have a lower incidence of akathisia. A variety of compounds have been reported effective for the treatment of akathisia including beta-adrenergic blockers, anticholinergic drugs, and benzodiazepines. There have also been reports on the use of clonidine for akathisia, but the evidence in its favor is scant, and clonidine has the additional problem of causing hypotension.

In the treatment of akathisia, various situations, calling for differing approaches, can arise. The authors recommend the following:

A. When the patient is treated with a high-potency antipsychotic drug and does not have other EPS
   1. First choice: a beta-adrenergic blocker, such as propranolol, 10–30 mg tid (nadolol can also be employed) (see Chapter 7)
   2. Second choice: an anticholinergic, such as benztropine, 2 mg bid
   3. Third choice: a benzodiazepine, such as lorazepam, 1 mg tid, or clonazepam, 0.5 mg bid
B. When the patient is treated with a low-potency antipsychotic drug (e.g., thioridazine) or an antipsychotic and a cyclic antidepressant and does not have other EPS
   1. First choice: propranolol, 10–30 mg tid
   2. Second choice: lorazepam, 1 mg tid, or clonazepam, 0.5 mg bid
   3. Third choice: benztropine, 1 mg bid (watch for additive anticholinergic toxicity)
C. When the patient is treated with an antipsychotic and manifests other EPS (dystonias or parkinsonism)

1. First choice: benztropine, 2 mg bid
2. Second choice: benztropine with propranolol, 10–30 mg tid
3. Third choice: benztropine with lorazepam, 1 mg tid, or clonazepam, 0.5 mg bid
D. When other EPS are present and akathisia is unresponsive to an anticholinergic alone
   1. First choice: benztropine, 2 mg bid, with propranolol, 10–30 mg tid
   2. Second choice: benztropine, 2 mg bid, with lorazepam, 1 mg tid, or clonazepam, 0.5 mg bid

Neuroleptic Malignant Syndrome

CLINICAL PRESENTATION. Neuroleptic malignant syndrome (NMS) is an extremely serious idiosyncratic reaction to neuroleptic drugs. The major symptoms of NMS are rigidity, fever, autonomic instability, and delirium. Symptoms usually develop over a period of several hours to several days with rigidity typically preceding fever and autonomic instability. Fever may be high, with temperatures of 41°C or higher commonly reported. Lead-pipe rigidity is typical, with increased muscle tone leading to myonecrosis in some cases. When patients are also dehydrated, the resulting myoglobinuria may be severe enough to cause renal failure. Autonomic symptoms include instability of blood pressure, often including both hyper- and hypotension, tachycardia, diaphoresis, and pallor. Cardiac arrhythmias may occur. In addition to rigidity, motor abnormalities including akinesia, tremor (which may fluctuate in severity), and involuntary movements have been reported. The patients are usually confused and often mute. There may be fluctuations in level of consciousness from agitation to stupor. Seizures or coma may also occur.

Neuroleptic malignant syndrome is a clinical diagnosis with a relatively wide continuum of severity. Since there are no clear criteria for making a diagnosis, especially in milder cases, it is difficult to state mortality rates. Although there are no specific laboratory findings, creatinine phosphokinase is usually elevated. For unknown reasons, liver function tests may also be abnormal, including elevations of transaminases and lactic dehydrogenase. The white blood cell count may also be slightly elevated.

Risk factors for development of NMS include dehydration, poor nutrition, external heat load, and possible intercurrent medical illness. Although all typical neuroleptics have been associated with NMS, there is evidence to suggest that high doses of high-potency neuroleptics increase the risk. Neuroleptic malignant syndrome has not been reported with clozapine as a single agent.

In severely psychotic patients, the following question often arises: Can the patient receive antipsychotics again after having had NMS? In fact, it appears that not all patients who have had NMS suffer a recurrence, even with the same drug that had previously caused the syndrome. Nonetheless, case reports accumulating in the literature suggest that a substantial percentage of patients who have developed NMS once, have a recurrence. Given the serious morbidity and possible lethality of this syndrome, it is prudent to withhold antipsychotics from patients who have had NMS unless there are compelling indications to resume this treatment and no alternative can be found. In such cases, the lowest possible doses of low-potency drugs, such as thioridazine, are probably the safest course. Ideally, treatment will not be resumed for at least 4 weeks after full resolution of NMS symptoms. The risks and benefits of such a decision should be fully discussed with the patient and, if appropriate, with his or her family.

TREATMENT. Meticulous supportive care is critical, including adequate hydration, use of cooling blankets for very high fever, turning of patients to avoid decubitus ulcers, cardiac monitoring, and monitoring of urine output and renal function. Should renal failure occur, dialysis may be necessary, but dialysis cannot be expected to remove antipsychotics because they are highly bound to plasma proteins and peripheral tissues. Specific treatments are experimental, but several have been used. Dantrolene, a direct-acting muscle relaxant, may decrease rigidity, secondary hyperthermia, and tachycardia. Response usually occurs quite rapidly. Dosages for this indication are not well established, but dosages in the range of 0.8–10.0 mg/kg/day have been advocated. In general, dosages of 1–3 mg/kg/day PO or IV, divided into a qid regimen, seem to be effective. Dosages above 10 mg/kg/day have been associated with hepatotoxicity. The dopamine agonist bromocriptine is thought to act centrally to decrease some of the symptoms of NMS. There are conflicting opinions on whether bromocriptine speeds recovery. Full response is said to require several days of treatment. Treatment with bromocriptine usually begins at 2.5 mg PO tid and is increased as tolerated to 5–10 mg PO tid. Dantrolene and bromocriptine can be administered together. The duration of therapy with either drug is not well established, but it is prudent to continue the drugs for a week after symptoms of NMS have passed.

Tardive Dyskinesia

Tardive dyskinesia is a syndrome of long-standing or permanent abnormal involuntary movements that is most commonly caused by the long-term use of typical antipsychotic (neuroleptic) drugs. At least 20% of patients who are treated with neuroleptic drugs long-term develop TD. Tardive dyskinesia presents clinically as involuntary movements of the tongue, facial, and neck muscles, upper and lower extremities, truncal musculature, or occasionally muscle groups that subserve breathing and swallowing. Buccolingual-masticatory movements are usually seen early in the course of the disorder and are characterized by tongue thrusting (often visible to the observer as the tongue pushing against the cheeks or lips), tongue protrusions, lip smacking, puckering of the lips, chewing movements, and cheek puffing. Excessive unnecessary facial movements including grimacing, blinking, and rapid ticlike movements of the face or periorbital musculature also can be seen in the early phases of TD. Although the movements may occasionally be difficult to distinguish from stereotyped posturing that may occur spontaneously in chronically psychotic individuals, TD generally appears less voluntary and usually has a more choreoathetoid quality.

Tardive dyskinesia rarely develops in patients who have had less than 3–6 months of antipsychotic drug exposure. The only firmly established risk factor for TD besides antipsychotic drug exposure is being over age 50, although there is some evidence that females may be at greater risk than males. There is inconsistent evidence that patients with mood disorders may be at greater risk for developing TD and that intermittent dosing (particularly among patients with mood disorders) may increase risk of TD. Presently, none of the standard antipsychotic drugs is known to be more or less likely to cause TD than another. Clozapine as a sole agent does not appear to be associated with TD. There is no clear correlation between development of parkinsonism while on antipsychotic drugs and the risk for TD. There is some suggestion that chronic use of anticholinergic compounds may increase the risk of TD; thus, their use should be minimized if possible.

Tardive dyskinesia often appears while the patient is still on medication. However, antipsychotic drugs can mask the symptoms of TD, and the abnormal involuntary movements may only become apparent on discontinuation or lowering of the drug dosage. When TD-like movements occur after a decrease in drug dosage or discontinuation and then regress over several days or weeks, they are defined as withdrawal dyskinesia. If relatively permanent, they are defined as TD. While there is no solid evidence to suggest that withdrawal dyskinesia portends TD if antipsychotics are resumed, it would be judicious to discontinue treatment with typical antipsychotic drugs if clinically possible. Treatment with clozapine could be considered as an alternative in this situation.

There is some disagreement in the literature on the long-term prognosis for TD among patients with TD who continue to receive typical antipsychotic drugs. Some investigators find progression of TD, but other investigations have found that once established, TD symptoms may reach a plateau or, in some cases, even improve. Pending additional research, the clinician must make a judgment in patients with serious psychotic disorders who are unable to take clozapine. It currently appears that if the psychotic disorder is serious, it may cause less morbidity to continue treatment, even with a typical antipsychotic drug, than to make TD the sole focus of the treatment. Clearly this clinical judgment requires a full discussion with the patient and family.

Tardive dystonia, a syndrome of late-onset refractory dystonias, has been reported uncommonly in schizophrenic patients treated chronically with typical antipsychotic drugs. There may be considerable overlap with TD. The natural history and risk factors are not well understood.

PREVENTION. There is no reliable treatment for TD. Thus, the optimal approach is to prevent it by limiting use of antipsychotic drugs to situations in which they are truly indicated. In particular, patients with mood, anxiety, or personality disorders should not be treated with antipsychotic drugs for protracted periods of time unless there is some compelling clinical evidence to show that the benefits outweigh the potential risks of developing TD. It is also judicious to avoid long-term use of antipsychotics whenever possible in the treatment of mental retardation, organic brain syndromes, or in the elderly, as these patients may be at particular risk for TD.

The clinician should examine all patients neurologically prior to initiating antipsychotic drug treatment. Optimally, a standardized scale for abnormal movements should be employed such as the *Abnormal Involuntary Movement Scale* (AIMS), published by the National Institute of Mental Health. These examinations should be repeated no less than every 6 months while the patient is on antipsychotic drugs. If treatment with an antipsychotic is required for 1 year, the clinician should attempt to taper or discontinue the drug and perform the neurologic evaluation at a lowered dosage of the

Table 2-7. Differential diagnosis of tardive dyskinesia

Neurologic disorders
  Wilson's disease
  Huntington's disease
  Brain neoplasms
  Fahr's syndrome
  Idiopathic dystonias (including blepharospasm, mandibular dystonia, facial "tics")
  Meige's syndrome (spontaneous oral dyskinesias)
  Torsion dystonia (familial disorder without psychiatric symptoms)
  Postanoxic or postencephalitic extrapyramidal symptoms
Drugs and other toxicities
  Antidepressants
  Lithium
  Anticholinergics
  Phenytoin
  L-Dopa and dopamine agonists
  Amphetamines and related stimulants
  Magnesium and other heavy metals

---

antipsychotic or while the patient is off the drug. If evidence of TD is noted, the clinician should discuss the implications with the patient and family, so that an informed decision can be made with regard to continuing the antipsychotic drug or switching to clozapine.

DIFFERENTIAL DIAGNOSIS. A variety of primary neurologic disorders are similar to TD (Table 2-7).

TREATMENT. Although many treatments including lithium, lecithin, physostigmine, and benzodiazepines have been tried, there is no consistently successful treatment for TD. There has been a recent report that clozapine treatment may decrease TD symptoms, but confirmation is needed.

Cardiac Toxicity

Pimozide and the low-potency antipsychotic drugs thioridazine and mesoridazine may slow cardiac conduction. Thus, they are mildly antiarrhythmic but can cause problems as well, including heart block and prolongation of the QTc with risk of torsades de pointes ventricular tachycardia. Although the toxicity of these drugs is most likely to be evident in overdose, it may occur in therapeutic doses as well. Patients with known cardiac disease should therefore be treated with high-potency agents. Risperidone has also been reported to increase the QTc.

The electrocardiogram (ECG) may show an increase in the QT and PR intervals, ST segment depression, and increased heart rate, all of which may be of little clinical consequence, except in patients who have underlying cardiac disease. QT prolongation beyond the normal range should prompt the physician to change to a different neuroleptic (e.g., haloperidol).

Clozapine is known to cause tachycardia independent of postural hypotension, which can be severe at times and may limit its use.

Postural Hypotension

Postural hypotension most commonly develops with the use of the lower-potency antipsychotic drugs, especially chlorpromazine, thioridazine, and clozapine. However, the high-potency drug risperidone also produces postural hypotension. This side effect is due to alpha-adrenergic receptor blockade by these compounds. Postural hypotension may be severe enough to cause syncope. Hypotension almost always improves when the patient is supine; patients should be warned to get up from recumbency slowly.

Ocular Side Effects

Blurred Vision

Because the low-potency agents such as chlorpromazine, thioridazine, mesoridazine, and clozapine are relatively anticholinergic, they may cause cycloplegia (the inability to accommodate). Patients may complain of blurred vision, usually with the greatest difficulty in reading. The medium-potency drugs (e.g., perphenazine) can occasionally cause this effect as well. In addition, blurred vision can be caused by anticholinergic compounds given to treat EPS. Often, reading glasses can correct the problem.

Glaucoma

Any anticholinergic drug may precipitate an attack of narrow-angle glaucoma; therefore, a history of glaucoma should prompt the use of a high-potency antipsychotic agent, avoidance of antiparkinsonians, and an ophthalmologic follow-up. Narrow-angle glaucoma is a medical emergency. Patients with open-angle glaucoma can be managed on neuroleptics if their glaucoma is concomitantly treated by an ophthalmologist.

Ocular Pigmentation

This side effect can be divided into two categories. Pigmentation of the lens, cornea, conjunctiva, and retina (often associated with skin pigmentation) is one category. This occurs mostly with the use of low-potency antipsychotics and is unlikely to interfere with vision except in extremely severe cases. The second category is pigmentary retinopathy, which is associated with the use of thioridazine above dosages of 800 mg/day and which leads to irreversible degenerative changes with visual impairment. Thioridazine should never be used at dosages above 800 mg/day for this reason. Patients on thioridazine with visual complaints should be examined by an ophthalmologist.

Cutaneous Side Effects

As with any class of drugs in medicine, the antipsychotics can cause allergic rashes, usually within the first 2 months of treatment. These are most commonly maculopapular erythematous rashes that affect the upper trunk, face, neck, and extremities. Although rashes are usually mild, exfoliative dermatitis has been reported. Discontinuation of the drug is followed by a remission of these symptoms. The physician should choose a compound from another chemical class if antipsychotic treatment is to be resumed.

Low-potency antipsychotics can act as photosensitizers, leading to severe sunburn. In addition, there are rare reports of blue-gray discoloration of the patient's skin, usually associated with ocular pigmentary changes. Although cosmetically undesirable, this effect has not been shown to predispose patients to further cutaneous pathology.

Hypothalamic and Pituitary Side Effects

The major endocrinologic effect of the typical antipsychotic compounds is hyperprolactinemia; the normal tonic dopaminergic inhibition of prolactin is blocked by all of the available antipsychotics except clozapine. In females this can result in galactorrhea (also seen rarely in males), amenorrhea, or both. In males, hyperprolactinemia may cause impotence. Because of its low affinity for D_2 dopamine receptors, clozapine has little or no effect on prolactin levels.

Although the effects are poorly understood, antipsychotics are known to predispose certain patients to **hyperthermia** or to marked **weight gain**, presumably by a hypothalamic mechanism. Severe neuroleptic-induced obesity may lead to drug refusal. There are several reports that molindone causes less obesity than the other antipsychotics.

Hepatic Side Effects

Antipsychotics, especially chlorpromazine, have been associated with cholestatic jaundice, probably secondary to a hypersensitivity reaction in certain predisposed individuals. This presents typically within the first 2 months of treatment and includes nausea, malaise, fever, pruritus, abdominal pain, and jaundice. Elevations of alkaline phosphatase and bilirubin accompanied by minor elevations of the transaminase are seen. Hepatitis should prompt discontinuation of the drug. The syndrome usually remits within 2–4 weeks after discontinuation. If further antipsychotic therapy is indicated, a different chemical class should be chosen.

Hematologic Side Effects

Agranulocytosis is a potentially life-threatening hematologic side effect seen most commonly with clozapine and very rarely with aliphatic and piperidine phenothiazine antipsychotics. The incidence with clozapine may be 1–3%. As emphasized previously, it is **imperative** to monitor white blood cell counts **weekly** for the entire treatment period with clozapine and for several weeks after discontinuation. A drop of 50% or a white blood cell count of below 3000 should lead to immediate discontinuation. With other antipsychotics it is better to instruct patients to report signs of infection (e.g., sore throats) than to monitor blood counts routinely. Symptomatic agranulocytosis requires immediate discontinuation of the medication. When agranulocytosis is associated with an antipsychotic drug in a particular patient, that drug must never be resumed.

OVERDOSAGE

Although the antipsychotic drugs have many toxicities that interfere with their therapeutic use, they have little potential for causing death if taken in overdose. Generally, the most serious complications of overdose are coma and hypotension, both of which should respond to volume expansion. Rarely, lethal cardiac arrhythmias may occur, probably most commonly with pimozide, thioridazine, and mesoridazine. These drugs may prolong the QT interval and precipitate heart block or torsades de pointes ventricular tachycardia. Whether risperidone will have similar problems in overdose is not yet known.

The more common manifestations of overdose may differ between high- and low-potency antipsychotics. Low-potency drugs such as chlorpromazine and thioridazine generally produce central nervous system (CNS) depression. Coma may result after 3–4 g of chlorpromazine. Low-potency drugs may also lower the seizure threshold markedly when taken in overdose, and thioridazine also has potent anticholinergic effects. In addition, these drugs have potent anti–alpha-adrenergic effects and may cause significant hypotension. Like all neuroleptics, these drugs may produce hypothermia or hyperthermia. Cardiac manifestations occur infrequently but may include QT prolongation and ventricular tachyarrhythmias, especially with thioridazine.

Higher-potency antipsychotic drugs can produce either CNS depression or CNS excitation with agitation, delirium, and severe extrapyramidal effects, such as muscular rigidity, tremor, or catatonic symptoms. Thermoregulation may also be impaired. Cardiac arrhythmias are rare but have been reported.

With serious overdoses, the basis of treatment is meticulous supportive care. Central nervous system excitation can be treated with low doses of lorazepam. Hypotension that does not respond to volume expansion will respond to vasopressors such as norepinephrine or phenylephrine. Beta-adrenergic agonists should be avoided because they may worsen vasodilatation. Hypothermia should be treated with slow warming. Hyperthermia should be treated with antipyretics and, if necessary, cooling blankets. Severe extrapyramidal effects should be treated with diphenhydramine, 50 mg IM or IV, or benztropine, 2 mg IM or IV. Because cardiac arrhythmias may occur, cardiac monitoring is necessary.

Ventricular tachyarrhythmias may be treated with lidocaine. Direct-current (DC) cardioversion is the treatment for life-threatening tachyarrhythmias. Torsades de pointes ventricular tachycardia, which may occur with pimozide, thioridazine, or mesoridazine, is best managed with isoproterenol or overdrive pacing.

If an ingestion was recent, induction of emesis (which may be difficult because of the antiemetic properties of the drug) or evacuation of the gastric contents through a nasogastric tube is indicated. After emesis is complete, administration of activated charcoal with a cathartic is helpful in adsorbing any remaining drug. Forced diuresis or dialysis is not helpful in removing antipsychotic drugs.

BIBLIOGRAPHY

Mechanism of Action

Hyman, S. E. How antipsychotic drugs might work. *Harvard Rev. Psychiatry* 1 : 68, 1993.

Van Tol, H. H., Bunzow, J. R., Guan, H. C., et al. Cloning of the gene for a human dopamine D_4 receptor with high affinity for the antipsychotic clozapine. *Nature* 350 : 610, 1991.

Schizophrenia and Other Psychotic Disorders

Baldessarini, R. J., and Davis, J. M. What is the best maintenance dose of neuroleptics in schizophrenia? *Psychiatry Res.* 3 : 115, 1980.

Kane, J., Rifkin, A., Quitkin, F., et al. Low dose fluphenazine decanoate in the maintenance treatment of schizophrenia. *Psychiatry Res.* 1 : 341, 1979.

Lerner, Y., Lwow, E., Levitan, A., and Belmacher, R. H. Acute high dose parenteral haloperidol treatment of psychosis. *Am. J. Psychiatry* 136 : 1061, 1979.

Meltzer, H. Y., Sommers, A. A., and Luchins, D. J. The effect of neuroleptics and other psychotropic drugs on negative symptoms in schizophrenia. *J. Clin. Psychopharmacol.* 6 : 329, 1986.

Other Psychiatric and Neurologic Disorders

Goldberg, S. C., Schulz, C., Schulz, P. M., et al. Borderline and schizotypal personality disorders treated with low-dose thiothixene vs. placebo. *Arch. Gen. Psychiatry* 43 : 680, 1986.

Pfeiffer, R. F., Kang, J., Graber, B., et al. Clozapine for psychosis in Parkinson's disease. *Movement Disorders* 5 : 239, 1990.

Ross, M. S., and Moldofsky, H. Comparison of pimozide with haloperidol in Gilles de la Tourette syndrome. *Lancet* 1 : 103, 1977.

Shapiro, E., Shapiro, A. K., Fulop, G., et al. Controlled study of haloperidol, pimozide, and placebo for the treatment of Gilles de la Tourette syndrome. *Arch. Gen. Psychiatry* 46 : 722, 1989.

Therapeutic Use

Levinson, D. F., Simpson, G. M., Singh, H., et al. Fluphenazine dose, clinical response, and extrapyramidal symptoms during acute treatment. *Arch. Gen. Psychiatry* 47 : 761, 1990.

Van Putten, T., Marder, S. R., and Mintz, J. A controlled dose comparison of haloperidol in newly admitted schizophrenic patients. *Arch. Gen. Psychiatry* 47 : 754, 1990.

Clozapine

Alvir, J. M. J., Lieberman, J. A., Safferman, A. Z., et al. Clozapine-induced agranulocytosis: Incidence and risk factors in the United States. *N. Engl. J. Med.* 329 : 162, 1993.

Kane, J., Honigfeld, G., Singer, J., and Meltzer, H. The Clozaril Collaborative Study Group: Clozapine for the treatment-resistant schizophrenic. A double-blind comparison vs. chlorpromazine/benztropine. *Arch. Gen. Psychiatry* 45 : 769, 1988.

Lieberman, J. A., Saltz, B. L., Johns, C. A., et al. The effects of clozapine on tardive dyskinesia. *Br. J. Psychiatry* 158 : 503, 1991.

McElroy, S. L., Dessain, E. C., Pope, H. G., et al. Clozapine in the treatment of psychotic mood disorders, schizoaffective disorder and schizophrenia. *J. Clin. Psychiatry* 52 : 411, 1991.

Meltzer, H. Y. Dimensions of outcome with clozapine. *Br. J. Psychiatry* 160(S) : 46, 1992.

Risperidone

Chouinard, G., Jones, B., Remington, G., et al. A Canadian Multicenter placebo-controlled study of fixed doses of risperidone and haloperidol in the treatment of chronic schizophrenic patients. *J. Clin. Psychopharmacol.* 13 : 25, 1993.

Marder, S. R., and Meibach, R. C. Risperidone in the treatment of schizophrenia. *Am. J. Psychiatry* 151 : 825, 1994.

Depot Antipsychotic Drugs

Kane, J. M. The use of depot neuroleptics: Clinical experience in the United States. *J. Clin. Psychiatry* 45(5, sec. 2) : 5, 1984.

Marder, S. R., van Putten, T., Mintz, J., et al. Costs and benefits of two doses of fluphenazine. *Arch. Gen. Psychiatry* 41 : 1025, 1984.

Side Effects and Toxicity

Arana, G. W., Goff, D., Baldessarini, R. J., and Keeper, G. The effect of anticholinergic prophylaxis on neuroleptic-induced dystonia. *Am. J. Psychiatry* 145 : 993, 1988.

Chouinard, G., Annable, L., Ross-Choiunard, A., et al. A 5-year prospective longitudinal study of tardive dyskinesia: Factors predicting appearance of new cases. *J. Clin. Psychopharmacol.* 8(S) : 21S, 1988.

Fleischhacker, W. W., Roth, S. D., and Kane, J. M. The pharmacologic treatment of neuroleptic-induced akathisia. *J. Clin. Psychopharmacol.* 10 : 12, 1990.

Fulop, G., Phillips, R. A., Shapiro, A. K., et al. ECG changes during haloperidol and pimozide treatment of Tourette's disorder. *Am. J. Psychiatry* 144 : 673, 1987.

Gardos, G., Casey, D. E., Cole, J. O., et al. Ten-year outcome of tardive dyskinesia. *Am. J. Psychiatry* 151 : 836, 1994.

Gelenberg, A. J., and Mandel, M. R. Catatonic reactions to high potency neuroleptic drugs. *Arch. Gen. Psychiatry* 34 : 947, 1977.

Levenson, J. L. Neuroleptic malignant syndrome. *Am. J. Psychiatry* 142 : 1137, 1985.

Pisciotta, A. V. Agranulocytosis induced by certain phenothiazine derivatives. *J.A.M.A.* 208 : 247, 1973.

Rosebush, P., and Stewart, T. A prospective analysis of 24 episodes of neuroleptic malignant syndrome. *Am. J. Psychiatry* 146 : 717, 1989.

Rosenberg, M. R., and Green, M. Neuroleptic malignant syndrome: Review of response to therapy. *Arch. Intern. Med.* 149 : 1927, 1989.

Drug Interactions

Goff, D. C., and Baldessarini, R. J. Drug interactions with antipsychotic agents. *J. Clin. Psychopharmacol.* 13 : 57, 1993.

Antipsychotic Drugs in Pregnancy

Ananth, J. Congenital malformations with psychopharmacologic agents. *Compr. Psychiatry* 16 : 437, 1975.

Ayd, F. J., Jr. Chlorpromazine 10 years' experience. *J.A.M.A.* 184 : 173, 1963.

3

Antidepressant Drugs

The antidepressant drugs are a heterogeneous group of compounds with major therapeutic effects in common—most importantly the treatment of major depressive illness. However, most of these drugs are also effective in the treatment of panic disorder and other anxiety disorders, and a subset are effective in the treatment of obsessive-compulsive disorder and a variety of other conditions (Table 3-1). For consideration of therapeutic spectrum of action and patterns of side effects, antidepressants are often subdivided into groups: **(1) selective serotonin reuptake inhibitors (SSRIs), (2) tricyclic and the related cyclic antidepressants (i.e., amoxapine and maprotiline), (3) monoamine oxidase inhibitors (MAOIs), and (4) other antidepressant compounds (bupropion, venlafaxine, trazodone, and nefazodone).** Because they overlap, the mechanisms of action and indications for use for the antidepressants are discussed together, but separate sections are provided for the method of administration and side effects.

MECHANISM OF ACTION

The precise mechanisms by which the antidepressant drugs exert their therapeutic effects remain unknown, although much is known about their acute actions within the nervous system. Their major interaction is with the monoamine neurotransmitter systems in the brain, particularly the norepinephrine and serotonin systems. Norepinephrine and serotonin are released throughout the brain by neurons originating in the locus ceruleus and brain stem raphe nuclei, respectively. Both of these neurotransmitters interact with multiple receptor types in the brain to regulate arousal, vigilance, attention, mood states, sensory processing, appetitive functions, and other global state functions.

Table 3-1. **Indications for antidepressants**

Effective
    Major depression (unipolar)
    Bipolar depression
    Prophylaxis against recurrence of major depression (unipolar)
    Panic disorder
    Depression with psychotic features in combination with an antipsychotic
    Bulimia
    Neuropathic pain (tricyclic drugs)
    Enuresis (imipramine best studied)
    Obsessive-compulsive disorder (clomipramine and SSRIs)
    Atypical depression (SSRIs or monoamine oxidase inhibitors)
Probably effective
    Attention-deficit/hyperactivity disorder
    Cataplexy due to narcolepsy
    Dysthymia (chronic depression)
    Organic mood disorders
    Pseudobulbar affect (pathologic laughing and weeping)
Possibly effective
    School phobia and separation anxiety

The importance of monoamine neurons in antidepressant action has been suggested by a number of observations. One of the classic animal models of depression utilizes the drug reserpine, which depletes neurons of monoamine neurotransmitters, including norepinephrine, serotonin, and dopamine. Similarly, reserpine has been shown to induce depression in some humans, which may be clinically indistinguishable from major depressive illness. In animal models, the cyclic antidepressants are partly able to reverse behavioral sedation induced by reserpine and other amine-depleting agents, such as tetrabenazine.

Norepinephrine, serotonin, and dopamine are removed from synapses after release by reuptake, mostly into presynaptic neurons. This mechanism of terminating neurotransmitter action is mediated by specific norepinephrine, serotonin, and dopamine reuptake transporter proteins. After reuptake, norepinephrine, serotonin, and dopamine are either reloaded into vesicles for subsequent release or broken down by the enzyme monoamine oxidase. The cyclic antidepressants and venlafaxine block the reuptake of norepinephrine and serotonin in varying ratios, thus potentiating their action (Fig. 3-1). The SSRIs have no significant effects on norepinephrine reuptake. Monoamine oxidase inhibitors may potentiate the action of biogenic amines by blocking their intracellular catabolism. Such observations initially suggested that antidepressants work by increasing noradrenergic and/or serotonergic neurotransmission, thus compensating for a postulated state of relative deficiency. However, this simple theory cannot fully explain the action of antidepressant drugs for a number of reasons. The most important of these include the lack of convincing evidence that depression is characterized by a state of inadequate noradrenergic or serotonergic neurotransmission. Indeed, many melancholic patients appear to have increased turnover of norepinephrine. Moreover, blockade of reuptake by the cyclic antidepressants and SSRIs and inhibition of monoamine oxidase by MAOIs occur rapidly (within hours) after drug administration, but antidepressants are rarely clinically effective prior to 3 weeks and may require 6 weeks or more.

These considerations have led to the idea that inhibition of monoamine reuptake or inhibition of monoamine oxidase by antidepressants is an initiating event. The actual therapeutic actions of antidepressants, however, result from slower adaptive responses within neurons to these initial biochemical perturbations. Research investigating slow-onset changes in neurons that might better reflect the time course of antidepressant action is under way. It has been found, for example, that chronic (> 2 weeks) treatment of rats with cyclic antidepressants or MAOIs is associated with a reduction in number (down-regulation) of beta$_1$-adrenergic receptors, accompanied by a decreased activation of adenylyl cyclase by norepinephrine. Many antidepressants also down regulate alpha$_2$-adrenergic receptors and have variable effects on 5-HT$_2$ serotonin receptors. Changes in receptor number must currently be seen as correlates of long-term administration (established largely in normal rat brain), not a likely therapeutic mechanism. There is no convincing theory to explain how monoamine receptor regulation could have an effect on mood disorders. Slow-onset changes in the nervous system that may be related convincingly to the mechanism of action of antidepressants are actively being sought. Important

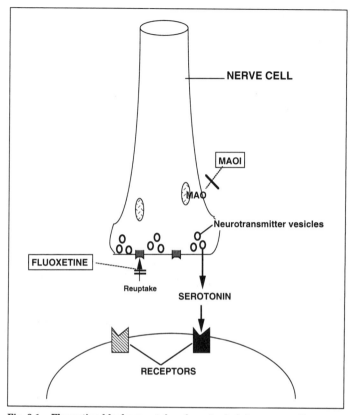

Fig. 3-1. Fluoxetine blocks reuptake of serotonin into presynaptic serotonin neurons by blocking the reuptake transporter protein. The action of monoamine neurotransmitters in the synapse is terminated by reuptake via specific reuptake transporters. The selective serotonin reuptake inhibitors, such as fluoxetine, specifically block the serotonin transporter; the tricyclics and venlafaxine block both the norepinephrine and serotonin transporters. The resulting increases in synaptic neuro-transmitters initiates slow adaptive responses that produce clinical improvement. MAOI = monoamine oxidase inhibitors.

candidates include antidepressant-induced changes in patterns of neuronal gene expression.

Although progress in understanding the mechanism of clinical action of antidepressants has been slow, receptor studies have been useful in understanding some of their side effects. For example, it has been found that the rank order of binding affinities of cyclic antidepressants at muscarinic cholinergic receptors generally parallels the potency of their clinical anticholinergic effects (e.g., amitriptyline > doxepin > imipramine > desipramine). Similarly, doxepin and amitriptyline have high affinities for histamine H_1 receptors, partially explaining their strong sedative effects (sedation is also a function of muscarinic receptor blockade). Such information is very useful in the pharmaceutical industry for screening compounds for possible clinical use.

INDICATIONS

Given the roles of norepinephrine and serotonin neurons in regulating global brain states, it is not surprising that, by interacting with these systems, certain antidepressant drugs can treat not only mood disorders, but also anxiety disorders, eating disorders, obsessive-compulsive disorder, and chronic pain syndromes. Additional uses are likely to be discovered. Indeed the term *antidepressant* is far too narrow and may raise issues in patient education when these drugs are prescribed for indications other than depression.

Since the introduction of fluoxetine, the SSRIs have become the most often prescribed initial treatment for major depression. The success of the SSRIs in displacing tricyclic drugs as first-choice agents is not based on established differences in efficacy for unselected populations, but rather on a generally more favorable side effect profile such as lack of anticholinergic and cardiac side effects, a high therapeutic index (ratio of lethal dose–therapeutic dose), and lower risk of withdrawal symptoms. Further, in certain subtypes of depression to be discussed subsequently and in obsessive-compulsive disorder, SSRIs offer advantages in efficacy over the tricyclics. Nonetheless, the tricyclic drugs remain important therapeutic options for the treatment of depression and anxiety disorders. Because of their toxicity and risk, MAOIs are a class of drug reserved for patients who have failed other treatments but are frequently effective when other drugs have failed. Drugs more recently introduced in the United States, venlafaxine and nefazadone, have side effects and safety advantages over the tricyclic antidepressants similar to the SSRIs; their place in the depression treatment algorithm is currently being defined by clinical experience.

Suicide Risk

The tricyclic and related cyclic antidepressants (maprotiline and amoxapine) and the MAOIs have a narrow therapeutic index, making them potentially lethal in overdose, unlike the SSRIs, trazodone, venlafaxine, nefazadone, and, despite its risk of seizures, bupropion. Thus, a careful evaluation of impulsiveness and suicide risk influences not only the decision as to the need for hospitalization but also the choice of an antidepressant, especially for those who will be treated as outpatients. For potentially suicidal or highly impulsive patients, the SSRIs, venlafaxine, nefazadone, trazodone, or potentially bupropion would be a better initial choice than a cyclic compound or MAOI. Patients at elevated suicide risk who cannot tolerate these safer compounds or who do not respond to them should not receive large quantities or refillable prescriptions for tricyclics or MAOIs. Generally, patients who are new to treatment or those at more than minimal risk for suicide whose therapeutic relationship is unstable should receive a limited supply of any medication.

Evaluation for suicide risk must continue even after the initiation of treatment. Suicidal thoughts and intentions may be slow to respond to treatment, and patients may become demoralized before therapeutic efficacy is evident. Side effects and, most importantly, intercurrent life events may trigger suicidal thoughts prior to a full therapeutic response. Thus, rarely, for a variety of reasons, patients may temporarily become more suicidal following the initiation of treatment. Should such worsening occur, appropriate interventions may include management of side effects, more frequent monitoring, discontinuation of the initial treatment, or hospitalization.

Major Depression

For patients who meet DSM-IV criteria for major depression, it can be expected that approximately 50% will fully recover with a single *adequate* trial (i.e., adequate dose for at least 6 weeks) of any effective antidepressant. Of the remainder, the majority will show some degree of improvement, but 10–15% will not improve substantially. For patients with comorbid psychiatric disorders such as personality disorders or psychotic disorders, the response rates will be lower. The best predictor of response to drug therapy is meeting the DSM-IV criteria regardless of the presence or absence of stressful antecedent life events. For those who do not recover fully, combined treatment or selection of another antidepressant will benefit the majority.

Based on controlled trials, as many as 20–40% of patients who improve to some degree may be exhibiting a placebo response. Placebo response, compared with true drug response, emerges earlier and is more variable. Therefore, loss of response early in the course may not represent loss of a true drug response and may indicate the need for more vigorous or prolonged treatment. Placebo response is less likely to occur with more severely depressed patients.

The most common reasons for failure of drug treatment are **inadequate drug dosage** and **inadequate length of drug trial.** Some clinicians continue to question whether, in general use, trazodone is as effective as the other approved antidepressants. Whether the newer related compound nefazodone will prove to have broader efficacy in general clinical settings remains to be seen. The majority of patients who fail adequate trials of drug therapy respond to electroconvulsive therapy (ECT). Recent studies have suggested that some forms of short-term psychotherapy (cognitive and interpersonal therapies) may be as effective as pharmacotherapy in milder depressions. The more serious the depression, the clearer the advantage of drug therapy over psychotherapies in terms of efficacy.

Subtypes of Depression

Even with the DSM-IV criteria, depression remains heterogeneous in its presentation and presumably in its etiology. Research on valid subtypes is in progress, but it is already possible to identify groups of patients with specific features that differentiate them from patients with simple major depression and may predict differential treatment responses.

Depressed Phase of Bipolar Disorder

The classification of depression into unipolar and bipolar is well supported by longitudinal, family, and treatment studies. All classes of antidepressants are effective in treating episodes of depression in patients with bipolar disorder. Unfortunately, these drugs also have certain liabilities in bipolar patients:

1. As many as 30–50% of bipolar patients may develop a manic episode during treatment with an antidepressant. Concomitant therapy with lithium or anticonvulsants may only be partially protective against this "switch" into mania.
2. In some bipolar patients, antidepressants may initiate and maintain rapid cycling (a state with more than three episodes or two or more continuous complete cycles per year, often characterized by diminished response to lithium).

Given these concerns, it is clinically useful for each bipolar patient to make a chart graphically representing periods of depression, hypomania, mania, and mixed symptoms over time as deflections up or down from a euthymic baseline. The medications employed should be recorded on this graphic time line as well. Such charting will help the clinician identify patterns of therapeutic efficacy and iatrogenically induced worsening should they occur.

If induction of mania occurs during antidepressant treatment, the antidepressant should be discontinued. If subsequent depressions occur, an antidepressant should be used for the shortest interval until symptoms improve and then treatment continued with lithium or anticonvulsants alone. There is preliminary evidence to suggest that bupropion may be less likely than tricyclic antidepressants to precipitate mania in rapid-cycling bipolar type II patients (i.e., patients with depressions and antidepressant-induced hypomania), although, like all antidepressants, it has been associated with the onset of mania in some patients. The switch into mania has been observed with all SSRIs; based on low rates of manic switch in clinical studies of paroxetine for depression, however, studies of paroxetine in known bipolar patients are being initiated. A small number of patients may develop severe manias with all antidepressants, despite lithium or anticonvulsant prophylaxis. For these patients, it may prove necessary to attempt to ride out milder depressions without antidepressants and to employ ECT for more severe episodes. However, even ECT may induce mania in a small number of patients. In general, chronic administration of antidepressants is best avoided, if possible, in bipolar patients.

Atypical Depression

Atypical depression historically has been used to refer to two different groups of depressed patients, generally classified as "A" or "V" type, the former referring to patients with prominent anxiety symptoms, including panic, and the latter referring to those with reversed vegetative signs, including hypersomnia and hyperphagia instead of insomnia and anorexia. As currently used, the term *atypical depression* refers to a group of patients with mood reactivity, who in addition report such symptoms as rejection sensitivity, hypersomnia, hyperphagia (e.g., carbohydrate craving), and prominent fatigue. These patients clearly respond better to MAOIs (phenelzine is best studied) than to tricyclics, although tricyclics are superior to placebo. Similarly, the SSRIs appear to be superior to tricyclics in this population; whether they are as effective as MAOIs remains to be determined. This form of depression tends to have onset at an early age and multiple recurrences; therefore, long-term treatment is likely to be necessary. Given their relative safety and ease of use, the SSRIs are preferred for an initial trial.

Hostile/Irritable

Past attempts to discern subtypes of major depression yielded a possible "hostile" depressive subtype. Recent work indicates that a fraction of outpatient depressives are predominantly irritable while depressed and manifest intermittent outbursts of anger or rage, which may be termed anger attacks. Anger attacks emerge abruptly with minimal provocation; they are associated with a paroxysm of autonomic arousal reminiscent of panic attacks but feature explosive verbal or physical anger, usually directed at close companions or family members. Anecdotal and systematically ascertained data suggest an important therapeutic role for antidepressants, especially SSRIs and MAOIs, in these patients.

Grief, Bereavement, and Loss

Following bereavement, loss of a job, or a life event leading to significant loss of self-esteem, individuals may experience symptoms of depression. It is important to distinguish depressive illness from normal grief or sadness. Although normally grieving individuals commonly sleep poorly and have decreased appetite, poor concentration, and other apparent neurovegetative symptoms immediately following the loss, these symptoms improve over several weeks' or months' time in the majority of cases. If depressive symptoms are particularly severe, persistent, or pervasive, are accompanied by serious suicidal thoughts or behavior, or are protracted beyond what might be expected for the precipitating stressor, psychiatric treatment is indicated.

In many cases the preferred treatment modality is psychotherapy aimed at helping the patient appropriately mourn the loss or develop adequate coping skills to deal with problems that have arisen. However, if the depressive symptoms are severe and unremitting, antidepressant therapy should be considered. Indeed, patients may be better able to utilize psychotherapy if their depressive symptoms are alleviated. Dosages are the same as for the treatment of major depression, although the treatment duration may be shorter, depending on the rapidity and completeness of the response.

Depression with Psychotic Features

Major depression accompanied by psychotic symptoms (e.g., delusions or hallucinations) responds poorly to treatment with antidepressants alone. Controlled studies demonstrate that depression with psychotic features is more effectively treated with the combination of an antidepressant and an antipsychotic drug (70–80% exhibiting significant improvement) than if treated with either class of drugs alone (30–50% response rate). Electroconvulsive therapy is at least as effective as the combined antidepressant-antipsychotic regimen and is the treatment of choice if this combination fails.

The recommended dosage of antipsychotic medication for depression with psychotic features has not been clearly established, but it appears that dosages slightly lower than those used in acute psychoses may be adequate, perhaps due to pharmacokinetic interactions with the antidepressant. Thus, patients might be started on 4–6 mg of haloperidol or the equivalent in addition to **full doses of an antidepressant,** with individual dosage adjustments as needed. The combination of low-potency antipsychotics (e.g., thioridazine, mesoridazine, or chlorpromazine) with tricyclic or related cyclic antidepressants is to be avoided because of additive anticholinergic toxicity and postural hypotension. Combinations of antipsychotics with SSRIs appear preliminarily to be effective. While diminishing the burden of anticholinergic, sedative, and hypotensive side effects, SSRIs may worsen the extrapyramidal side effects of antipsychotic drugs. Because of their relatively greater potential to inhibit the hepatic metabolism of drugs metabolized by the P450 2D6 isoenzyme, fluoxetine and paroxetine are more likely than sertraline or fluvoxamine to produce increases in antipsychotic drug levels and thus side effects or toxicity. Fixed combinations (e.g., Triavil) do not allow the clinician to adjust medications individually and therefore are not recommended. For this reason we also do not recommend amoxapine, an antidepressant with metabolites possessing some neuroleptic effects, which has also been reported effective for depression with psychotic features.

The anticholinergic effects of many tricyclic antidepressants are often sufficient prophylaxis against extrapyramidal symptoms; thus, additional anticholinergics should not routinely be prescribed when tricyclics are part of the combination. If additional anticholinergic medication proves necessary for extrapyramidal symptoms, careful monitoring for anticholinergic toxicity is important.

A more subtle clinical point is that antipsychotic drugs may themselves cause masked facies, akinesia, and blunting of affect, which can be confused with depressive symptoms; thus, other target symptoms, such as sleep, guilt, or psychotic symptoms, may be better indicators of improvement when patients are on combined antipsychotic-antidepressant regimens.

Given the serious morbidity and high suicide risk of depression with psychotic features, maintenance treatment must be considered. However, there are few data to guide the decision whether to continue with combined treatment or either agent alone. For a patient who continues well, general clinical wisdom is to discontinue the antipsychotic drug first, while maintaining the antidepressant treatment longer term.

Depression Comorbid with Other Disorders

Depression with Anxiety

Anxiety symptoms including panic attacks commonly accompany major depression. Patients with prominent anxiety symptoms are still likely to respond to antidepressant medication.

Many clinicians administer adjunctive benzodiazepines for symptomatic relief of anxiety in depressed patients. Adjunctive benzodiazepines offer initial relief of anxiety symptoms prior to onset of antidepressant efficacy. They may also be useful for residual symptoms that do not improve with the antidepressant (see Chap. 6). Because of its delayed onset of efficacy, buspirone cannot be used to provide initial relief. It is important to recognize that anti-depressants are the essential therapeutic agents in these cases and that full antidepressant doses are needed whether or not a benzodi-azepine produces initial improvements in such symptoms as anxiety and insomnia.

Depression Complicating Borderline Personality Disorder

There are generally two types of clinical situations in which anti-depressants are used in patients with borderline personality dis-order: (1) intercurrent major depression and (2) the presence of chronic depressive symptoms that are either two few in number or too mild to meet criteria for major depression.

Both typical and atypical major depression frequently complicate the course of borderline personality disorder. In general, the pres-ence of a personality disorder predicts a worse treatment outcome than expected for uncomplicated major depression; however, anti-depressants are still superior to placebo. Because these patients are often impulsive, angry, and self-destructive, first-choice medica-tions would be those that are less dangerous in overdose, for exam-ple, the SSRIs.

Some patients with borderline personality disorder have perva-sive depressive symptoms without meeting DSM-IV criteria for major depression or dysthymia. These patients may benefit from a trial of an antidepressant, particularly an SSRI or MAOI. Because of their difficulty of use, prescription of MAOIs in this population requires a strong alliance with the patient and great care.

In clinical studies, SSRIs improve not only depressive symptoms but also anger and hostility. In contrast, in one report, the tricyclic compound amitriptyline produced worsening in a significant num-ber of patients in self-destructive episodes and global ratings.

Depression Comorbid with Substance Abuse

Secondary depression often occurs in the context of alcohol abuse and abuse of other central nervous system (CNS) depressants (e.g., barbiturates). Most often, the depressive symptoms are due to direct toxic effects of the alcohol; therefore, the primary treatment should be detoxification. Given the possibilities of drug interactions with alcohol or barbiturates (including altered pharmacokinetics and possible additive CNS depression), prescription of antidepressants to active alcoholics should be avoided if possible. Generally, anti-depressants are indicated only if serious depressive symptoms per-sist for 4 weeks after successful detoxification or if the history indicates that mood disorder may be primary and not secondary to substance abuse.

In contrast, there is interest in the possibility that antidepres-sants may help maintain abstinence from cocaine. In particular, there are reports that desipramine has modest efficacy in reducing cocaine craving and increasing cocaine abstinence during the months following cessation of cocaine use.

Refractory Depression

A large number of patients respond partially or not at all to an initial antidepressant trial. It is important to ensure that the initial diagnosis was correct and that there is not an unsuspected comorbid condition (e.g., alcoholism or thyroid disease) impairing treatment response. There are three general strategies for treating refractory depression that can be employed in an orderly fashion (these strategies are discussed in detail for each specific class of drug):

1. **Optimization**: ensuring adequate drug doses for the individual, which may be higher than usual doses (e.g., fluoxetine, 40–80 mg; desipramine, 200–300 mg), and adequate duration of treatment (6 weeks or longer).
2. **Augmentation or combination**: addition of adjunctive lithium, L-triiodothyronine (T_3), or other drugs to an established antidepressant regimen.
3. **Substitution**: change in the primary drug, usually to an agent from a different drug class; for example, if the first drug was an SSRI, switch to a tricyclic. If, however, the first drug failed because of side effects, a drug within the initial class may be effective if it is tolerated. If the second trial fails and the patient remains seriously depressed, consideration should be given to the relative risks of a trial with a third medication (based on severity of symptoms and concern about time delay) versus the use of ECT.

Continuation and Maintenance Treatment

Based on studies with tricyclic antidepressants, patients with unipolar depression are at high risk for relapse if treatment is discontinued within the first 16 weeks of therapy. Therefore, in treatment responders, most experts favor a continuation of therapy for a minimum period of 6 months. Risk of recurrence, that is, the development of a new episode, is particularly elevated in patients with a chronic course before recovery, multiple prior episodes (three or more), or a first episode in late life. For these individuals, the optimal duration of maintenance treatment is unknown but is measured in years. Based on research to date, prophylactic efficacy of antidepressants has been observed for as long as 5 years with clear benefit. In contrast to the initial expectation that maintenance therapy would be effective at dosages lower than that required for acute treatment, the current consensus is that full-dose therapy is required for effective prophylaxis.

In the past, maintenance treatment was difficult because some tricyclic side effects increased or emerged over time, such as weight gain, dental caries, and continuation of such unpleasant sensations and symptoms as dry mouth and constipation. With newer drugs, especially the SSRIs, maintenance therapy is easier. Fluoxetine, sertraline, and paroxetine have all been found to remain effective for at least 1 year. There have been patients, however, treated with each of the classes of antidepressants for whom the drug has lost efficacy over time. In such patients, the same treatment strategies described for refractory depression are appropriate.

In a very small number of patients on SSRIs, apathy has emerged as a side effect that can be mistaken for recurrent depression. Apathy in the absence of associated depressive symptoms should prompt a decrease rather than an increase in the dosage.

Except for amoxapine, which possesses some neuroleptic properties and has been implicated in tardive dyskinesia, there are no known adverse effects specifically due to long-term antidepressant treatment. It should be recognized, however, that long-term experience with some of the newer compounds is limited.

Dysthymia

Dysthymia is heterogeneous clinically and likely heterogeneous in etiology. Seventy percent of dysthymic patients have a comorbid medical or psychiatric disorder. This disorder may have profound consequences for quality of life and for effective functioning in multiple life roles; this morbidity is more reflective of the duration of dysthymia than of the number of symptoms. An older belief that this class of patients would not respond to antidepressants may have reflected the mistaken idea that patients with "milder" symptoms would require only low doses of antidepressants, leading to inadequate dosing or duration of treatment. More recent studies of dysthymia treatment with SSRIs and tricyclics indicate that this is a treatment-responsive condition; moreover, the benefit of treatment is maintained with continued therapy as in major depression. Inasmuch as one cannot predict ahead of time which dysthymic patients will respond to antidepressant treatment, and given the safety and possible effectiveness of the SSRIs, a therapeutic trial should be considered for dysthymic patients. A therapeutic trial is particularly appropriate when there is

1. Presence of clear neurovegetative symptoms (e.g., sleep disorder, change in appetite, loss of energy, or diurnal variation in mood)
2. Prior history of mania
3. Family history of mood disorder
4. History of prior response to antidepressant drugs

Secondary Mood Disorders

Many medical illnesses and medications can produce secondary depressive syndromes (Table 3-2). When the depression is due to a treatable disorder or medication, it may remit with appropriate medical care or discontinuation of the offending drug. If, however, the depression is severe and does not remit within several weeks after treatment of the medical condition, it would be reasonable to initiate antidepressant therapy. For patients whose primary disorder has been treated, antidepressants can usually be discontinued soon after the depressive symptoms remit, although if depressive symptoms recur, the antidepressant therapy should probably be continued for 6 months as if the depression were primary.

Table 3-2.   Organic etiologies of depression

Drug induced: Reserpine, beta-blockers, alpha-methyldopa, levodopa, estrogens, corticosteroids, cholinergic drugs, benzodiazepines, barbiturates and similarly acting drugs, ranitidine, calcium channel blockers

Related to drug abuse: Alcohol abuse, sedative-hypnotic abuse, cocaine and other psychostimulant withdrawal

Metabolic disorders: Hyperthyroidism (especially in the elderly), hypothyroidism, Cushing's syndrome, hypercalcemia, hyponatremia, diabetes mellitus

Neurologic disorders: Stroke, subdural hematoma, multiple sclerosis, brain tumors (especially frontal), Parkinson's disease, Huntington's disease, uncontrolled epilepsy, syphilis, dementias, closed head injuries

Nutritional disorders: Vitamin B_{12} deficiency, pellagra

Other: Pancreatic carcinoma, viral infections (especially mononucleosis and influenza)

Certain neurologic disorders that have no definitive treatment (e.g., stroke, Parkinson's disease, Huntington's disease) commonly produce secondary depression. Stroke patients, in particular, develop secondary depression with an incidence greater than would be predicted by the degree of disability. Aggressive treatment of the depression may improve the patient's quality of life and his or her ability to participate in rehabilitation. For patients with depression secondary to an untreatable medical or neurologic illness, the duration of therapy must be determined empirically. Many patients with brain injuries or neurodegenerative disorders (e.g., Alzheimer's disease) manifest elevated susceptibility to the side effects of psychotropic medications.

Panic Disorder

The core manifestation of panic disorder is recurrent unexpected panic attacks. In addition, a substantial proportion of patients with panic disorder develop anticipatory anxiety and phobic avoidance, which may prove more disabling than the panic attacks themselves. When severe, phobic avoidance in the form of agoraphobia (fear of situations in which it may be difficult to gain help or escape) may cause patients to become entirely housebound. Tricyclic antidepressants, MAOIs, and high-potency benzodiazepines (alprazolam and clonazepam; see Chap. 6) have established efficacy in the treatment of panic attacks. Because of their side effect profile, the SSRIs are increasingly the first choice among the antidepressants for panic disorder, although systematic confirmatory data are still accumulating. One disadvantage of the SSRIs, similar to what is seen with the tricyclics, but unlike the MAOIs or benzodiazepines, is the risk of increased jitteriness and anxiety at the initiation of treatment. Thus SSRIs or tricyclics should initially be prescribed at the lowest daily doses possible (e.g., sertraline, 25 mg; paroxetine, 10 mg; fluoxetine, 2–5 mg; imipramine, 10 mg). Doses of fluoxetine under 10 mg require use of the liquid formulation or dissolving the contents of a capsule in juice or water and aliquoting the juice. Among the tricyclic antidepressants, imipramine is the best studied, although it is likely that all of the tricyclics are effective. As with other disorders, MAOIs may be the most effective of all but are reserved for treatment-refractory patients because of their side effects and difficulty of use.

Generally, the anticipatory anxiety and phobic avoidance observed in panic disorder respond slowly to antidepressant monotherapy. Therefore, cognitive behavior therapy is often used in conjunction with drug treatment.

Comorbid depression is very common in panic disorder; its presence requires the selection of antidepressant treatment rather than a benzodiazepine as the primary treatment for both disorders. For panic disorder uncomplicated by depression or for residual anxiety symptoms, many clinicians use a high-potency benzodiazepine. The major advantage of an antidepressant is low risk of dependence and therefore less difficulty with discontinuation (see Chap. 6). The major disadvantages are delayed onset, more side effects, and rather less efficacy for anticipatory anxiety.

Obsessive-Compulsive Disorder

Obsessive-compulsive disorder (OCD) involves recurrent intrusive thoughts that the patient recognizes as products of his or her own mind (obsessions) and/or repetitive, seemingly purposeful behavior designed to prevent or neutralize some dreaded consequence (compulsions). Of the drugs presently available in the United States, only clomipramine and the SSRIs appear to have significant anti-obsessional activity based on controlled studies and clinical experience. Approximately 50% of patients receiving an adequate trial of one of these medications improve. It is striking that all of these drugs have potent and relatively selective effects on inhibition of serotonin reuptake (although the major metabolite of clomipramine has significant effects on norepinephrine reuptake as well).

There have been smaller studies and case reports of positive anti-obsessional responses with many other drugs including tricyclic antidepressants (e.g., imipramine, desipramine, amitriptyline, and doxepin), MAOIs, and high-potency benzodiazepines, but these drugs have not proved reliably effective in large numbers of patients. Based on anecdotal evidence, MAOIs may be particularly effective for patients whose OCD is complicated by panic attacks, social phobia, or severe generalized anxiety. While benzodiazepines are not generally effective in treating OCD, clonazepam did prove superior to placebo in one controlled trial. Since obsessions may be quite bizarre, patients are at risk for inappropriate diagnosis of psychosis and treatment with antipsychotic drugs. The use of antipsychotic drugs in the treatment of well-diagnosed obsessions should be restricted to nonresponders to standard treatment who have accompanying schizotypal features or clinically significant tics.

Psychopharmacologic treatment is most effective in treating obsessions. Patients presenting with predominantly compulsive rituals often respond better to behavior therapy, including exposure (e.g., getting the patient to handle a feared source of contamination) and response prevention (e.g., not allowing the patient to perform a ritual for a certain period of time). For many patients, a combination of pharmacotherapy and behavior therapy will prove optimal.

For OCD, clomipramine is typically used in doses of 150–250 mg/day. Its use is limited by its anticholinergic effects. At doses above 250 mg/day there is also a relatively high incidence of seizures. Treatment of OCD with SSRIs also requires higher doses than are typically recommended for depression. For fluoxetine, doses of 60–80 mg/day are commonly required. Dosages as high as 120 mg/day are presently under study. Among the other SSRIs, there are preliminary clinical data that sertraline may be somewhat less effective for OCD than fluoxetine, paroxetine, and fluvoxamine.

Symptoms of OCD respond more slowly than symptoms of major depression. Thus trials of each medication should last for at least 12 weeks. Clomipramine at an average dose of 180 mg/day (range 100–250 mg/day) has also been reported to be effective in the treatment of trichotillomania (hair pulling), a condition hypothesized to be related to OCD. In this same study, desipramine was not effective (Swedo et al., 1989). Trichotillomania is difficult to treat in clinical practice.

Body Dysmorphic Disorder
Body dysmorphic disorder, sometimes referred to as dysmorphophobia, involves preoccupation with an imagined physical defect. Antipsychotic drugs, most notably pimozide and haloperidol, have been used in the past and produced only modest benefit. More recently SSRIs have been employed in high (OCD-like) doses,

preliminarily giving more satisfactory responses than antipsychotic drugs.

Posttraumatic Stress Disorder

Following an extremely traumatic experience, such as rape, severe abuse, or combat, posttraumatic stress disorder (PTSD) may develop, which includes nightmares about the event, a heightened startle reflex, sudden feelings of reexperiencing the traumatic event (flashbacks), and avoidance of objects or situations that are reminders of the event. Such symptoms may be disabling in themselves and may lead to further impairment secondary to avoidant behaviors. Fully effective treatments for the core symptoms of PTSD are lacking. When used in combination with psychosocial treatment, some patients have a partial or marked benefit from antidepressants, including MAOIs or SSRIs.

Social Phobia

Social phobia is defined as a persistent fear of social situations in which the individual feels open to scrutiny or humiliation. Several studies have identified MAOIs, specifically phenelzine and tranylcypromine, as potentially effective in reducing these fears and secondary avoidant behaviors (see also Chap. 6). Preliminary studies also support the use of SSRIs. Presently, cognitive and behavioral therapies are better established, but pharmacologic treatment for social phobia is an active area of research.

Bulimia

Several open and controlled trials support the use of SSRIs (fluoxetine is best studied), tricyclics, and MAOIs in the treatment of bulimia. Given the impulsiveness of these patients and the dangers of dietary indiscretions with MAOIs, this class of drugs is generally reserved for treatment-refractory patients who are nonetheless compliant with treatment. Bupropion also appears to be effective, but because of a high incidence of seizures in one study of bulimics, its use is not recommended in this disorder. Antidepressants produce improvement in binge frequency, vomiting and other purging, and attitude toward eating. In a multicenter placebo-controlled, double-blind trial of fluoxetine for bulimia, a dose of 60 mg/day was superior to 20 mg/day, which was in turn superior to placebo. These data and clinical experience suggest that higher doses of SSRIs than are typically used for depression may be required to treat bulimia. Because higher doses of SSRIs are safer and better tolerated than higher doses of cyclic antidepressants, SSRIs have become the first-choice pharmacologic treatment for bulimia. Although many responsive patients who have been studied in antidepressant trials had depressive symptoms, many did not. Pharmacotherapy should generally be part of a comprehensive treatment program.

Antidepressants appear to be far less successful in treating anorexia nervosa than bulimia, although a prior history of anorexia nervosa does not seem to influence antidepressant response among current bulimics.

Attention-Deficit/Hyperactivity Disorder

Attention-deficit/hyperactivity disorder begins in childhood with symptoms of difficulty paying attention, impulsiveness, and hyperactivity. Although it is most frequently treated with psychostimulants (see Chap. 7), some controlled trials have found the tricyclics imipramine and desipramine to be as effective as methylphenidate in treating the behavioral and cognitive disturbances associated with this disorder. Imipramine and desipramine have been used in dosages of 2–5 mg/kg/day. The advantage of antidepressants is once daily dosing; the disadvantage is that they have greater toxicity (e.g., anticholinergic and cardiac effects). Preliminary evidence suggests a role for bupropion in this condition as well. Reports of sudden death in children treated with desipramine clearly favors the use of psychostimulants as first-line drugs in this population.

Chronic Pain Syndromes

Tricyclic antidepressants have been shown to be effective in a variety of chronic pain syndromes, even in the absence of diagnosable major depression, and often at lower doses than those used for depression. For example, in the treatment of neuropathic pain, analgesic effects of amitriptyline have been demonstrated at blood levels lower than those thought to be antidepressant (analgesia at levels > 120 ng/ml; antidepressant at levels > 225 ng/ml) and at earlier times (1–2 weeks after initiation of therapy). In animal studies, imipramine and amitriptyline both have been shown to potentiate morphine analgesia and to possess analgesic properties themselves.

Clinically, tricyclic antidepressants are indicated for treatment of chronic pain syndromes, especially neuropathic pain (e.g., diabetic neuropathy, postherpetic neuralgia, or trigeminal neuralgia). Empirical trials in patients with tension headaches, back pain, and other chronically painful conditions are occasionally successful. Imipramine and amitriptyline have been the most widely prescribed antidepressants for the treatment of chronic pain syndromes; however, a recent study demonstrated equivalent efficacy of desipramine to amitriptyline. In the same study, and in general clinical practice, fluoxetine appeared to be ineffective. Because of its preferable side effect profile, patients might be started on desipramine. If low doses (e.g., 100–150 mg) are unsuccessful, higher doses (150–300 mg) might be prescribed if the patient has significant depressive symptoms. Patients who fail with desipramine might be tried on imipramine or amitriptyline before this class of drugs is abandoned.

Tricyclics, especially amitriptyline, also have been studied in migraine prophylaxis, with mixed results. Although some trials have found amitriptyline to be superior to placebo, it appears to be less effective than propranolol for migraine prophylaxis.

Facilitation of the actions of norepinephrine and perhaps serotonin in the dorsal horn of the spinal cord is thought to form the basis of the analgesic properties of tricyclic drugs. The relative ineffectiveness of fluoxetine even at the relatively high dose of 40 mg/day has, along with recent neuroanatomic data, raised questions about the role of serotonin in analgesia.

CHOICE OF ANTIDEPRESSANT

There are currently a large number of antidepressants available (Table 3-3), including the SSRIs, tricyclic and related compounds, the MAOIs, and other compounds (bupropion, venlafaxine, nefazadone, trazodone). Successful use of antidepressants requires

1. Good patient selection as determined by a thorough diagnostic evaluation

Table 3-3. Available preparations

Drug	Dosage Forms (mg)	Usual Daily Dose (mg/day)	Extreme Dose (mg/day)	Therapeutic Plasma Levels (ng/ml)
Selective serotonin reuptake inhibitors				
Fluoxetine (Prozac)	C: 10, 20 LC: 20 mg/5 ml	20	5–80	
Fluvoxamine (Luvox)	T: 20, 30	150–200	50–300	
Paroxetine (Paxil)	T: 20, 30	20	10–50	
Sertraline (Zoloft)	T: 50, 100	100–150	50–200	
Cyclic compounds				
Imipramine (Tofranil and generics)	T: 10, 25, 50 C: 75, 100, 125, 150 INJ: 25 mg/2 ml	150–200	50–300	> 225[a]
Desipramine (Norpramin and generics)	T: 10, 25, 50, 75, 100, 150 C: 25, 50	150–200	50–300	> 125
Amitriptyline (Elavil and generics)	T: 10, 25, 50, 75, 100, 150 INJ: 10 mg/ml	150–200	50–300	> 120 (?)[b]
Nortriptyline (Pamelor and generics)	C: 10, 25, 50, 75 LC: 10 mg/5 ml	75–100	25–150	50–150
Doxepin (Adapin, Sinequan, and generics)	C: 10, 25, 50, 75, 100, 150 LC: 10 mg/ml	150–200	25–300	100–250 (?)
Trimipramine (Surmontil)	C: 25, 50, 100	150–200	50–300	
Protriptyline (Vivactil)	T: 5, 10	15–40	10–60	
Maprotiline (Ludiomil)	T: 25, 50, 75	100–150	50–200	
Amoxapine (Asendin)	T: 25, 50, 100, 150	150–200	50–300	
Clomipramine (Anafranil)	C: 25, 50,75	150–200	50–250	

Other compounds			
Bupropion (Wellbutrin)	T: 75, 100	200–300	100–450
Venlafaxine (Effexor)		75–225	75–375
Trazodone (Desyrel and generics)	T: 50, 100, 150, 300	200–300	100–600
Nefazodone		200–300	100–600
Monoamine oxidase inhibitors			
Phenelzine (Nardil)	T: 15	45–60	15–90
Tranylcypromine (Parnate)	T: 10	30–50	10–90

C = capsules; INJ = injectable form; LC = liquid concentrate or solution; T = tablets.
[a]Sum of imipramine plus desipramine.
[b]Sum of amitriptyline plus nortriptyline.

2. Choice of a drug with a tolerable side effect profile for the given patient
3. Adequate dosage
4. Drug trial of at least 4 weeks, preferably 6 weeks for depression or panic disorder, and at least 12 weeks for OCD

Many patients with potentially treatable depression or panic disorder fail to improve because of inadequate dosing or duration of treatment or both.

As in the case of antipsychotic drugs, physicians do not routinely prescribe all antidepressants on the market, but it is useful for the clinician to be comfortable prescribing several drugs in each class that differ in side effects. The most important considerations in choosing among these drugs are efficacy and side effects. The efficacy of the available antidepressants for major depression, including various subtypes, and for other disorders is described under Indications. While there are some differences in efficacy across the class of antidepressants for subtypes of depression and for OCD, the major clinically significant differences among the antidepressants are in their side effects. All of the tricyclic antidepressants and related compounds (maprotiline and amoxapine) cause some degree of anticholinergic side effects and postural hypotension, and all are potentially cardiotoxic in susceptible individuals or in overdose (Table 3-4). The SSRIs, bupropion, venlafaxine, nefazodone, and trazodone lack the anticholinergic side effects and potential cardiotoxicity of the tricyclics. Trazodone produces sedation, postural hypotension, and nausea. The SSRIs and venlafaxine may cause agitation, insomnia, nausea, headache, and sexual dysfunction, among other side effects, but are generally more tolerable to patients than the older cyclic compounds. The MAOIs may cause significant side effects, including postural hypotension, and require dietary precautions.

At a minimum, general physicians should be comfortable prescribing at least two of the SSRIs, and at least one of the tricyclics that has a lower anticholinergic potency (e.g., nortriptyline or desipramine). Because psychiatrists will often be called upon to treat patients who have failed initial treatments, they should have broader experience, including experience with bupropion and MAOIs. The following are general guidelines for choosing an antidepressant:

1. It is reasonable to prescribe any drug that was clearly effective in the past if it was well tolerated by the patient.

2. Avoid drugs (e.g., amitriptyline, protriptyline) with the highest levels of anticholinergic activity to maximize patient comfort and compliance. (Despite its high anticholinergic potency, clomipramine is useful because of its efficacy in treating OCD.)

3. For patients with initial insomnia, some clinicians select a more sedating compound (e.g., imipramine) given at bedtime. To avoid anticholinergic and cardiovascular side effects, however, an alternative would be **temporary** use of a benzodiazepine combined with an SSRI. The sedating tricyclic drug amitriptyline has long been popular with physicians, but because it is among the most anticholinergic of the tricyclics, it should not be a first-choice agent. Trazodone, which lacks anticholinergic side effects, is very sedating, but its broad efficacy is questioned by some clinicians. Trazodone, 50 mg hs, has been used by some clinicians in place of a benzodi-

**Table 3-4.   Sedative, anticholinergic,
and hypotensive effects of antidepressants**

Class	Drug	Sedative Potency	Anti-cholinergic Effects	Orthostatic Hypotensive Effects
Cyclic drugs[a]	Amitriptyline	High	High	High
	Amoxapine	Low	Low	Moderate
	Clomipramine	High	High	High
	Desipramine	Low	Low	High
	Doxepin	High	High	Moderate
	Imipramine	Moderate	Moderate	High
	Maprotiline	Moderate	Low	Moderate
	Nortriptyline	Low	Low	Lowest tricyclic
	Protriptyline	Low	High	Low
	Trimipramine	High	Moderate	Moderate
SSRIs	Fluoxetine	Low	Absent	Very low
	Fluvoxamine	Low	Absent	Very low
	Paroxetine	Low	Absent	Very low
	Sertraline	Low	Absent	Very low
Miscellaneous compounds	Venlafaxine	Low	Absent	[b]
	Bupropion	Low	Absent	Very low
	Nefazodone	Moderate	Absent	Low
	Trazodone	High	Absent	Moderate
MAOIs	Phenelzine	Low	Very low	High
	Tranylcypromine	Low	Very low	High

[a]All of the tricyclic and related cyclic compounds have well-established cardiac arrhythmogenic potential.
[b]Venlafaxine may cause dose-dependent sustained increases in blood pressure in some patients.

azepine to treat initial insomnia in patients treated for depression with an SSRI. For most depressed patients, if insomnia is related to depression, the sleep difficulties will improve with any effective antidepressant over time, even those without sedation as a side effect. With more sedating drugs, on the other hand, the side effect may persist long after it is helpful and may interfere with patient function, well-being, and compliance.

4. Imipramine is available generically and has the advantage of being the least costly and best studied of all the tricyclics. It is, however, moderately anticholinergic and sedating, and has the other drawbacks of the tricyclics in terms of side effects.

5. For patients who want to avoid sedation, an SSRI, bupropion, or venlafaxine is a good choice. Among the tricyclics, desipramine and nortriptyline are usually not sedating.

6. In elderly patients, especially those with constipation or glaucoma, and in males with prostatic hypertrophy, the least anticholinergic drugs should be used, such as an SSRI, bupropion, or venlafaxine. Among the tricyclics, desipramine and nortriptyline have lower but still significant anticholinergic potency.

7. The SSRIs, bupropion, and venlafaxine do not cause postural hypotension. Nortriptyline may have an advantage among the tricyclics in causing relatively less postural hypotension than the others (although this observation has been debated).

8. In patients with serious delays in cardiac conduction, the SSRIs, bupropion, and venlafaxine are clearly preferable to the tricyclic compounds, amoxapine, or maprotiline. Electroconvulsive therapy is also safe in this population.

9. Epileptic patients may develop a primary depressive disorder or secondary depression. Because all of the tricyclic and related cyclic antidepressants and bupropion may decrease the seizure threshold, the use of an SSRI or MAOI is preferable. Trazodone also appears to have little effect on the seizure threshold. Clinical experience with venlafaxine and nefazodone in epileptic patients is limited. If tricyclic compounds must be used, for reasons of side effects or efficacy in a particular patient, adjustments may have to be made in ongoing antiepileptic treatments. When combining any antidepressant with an anticonvulsant, the clinician must be alert for pharmacokinetic interactions.

10. Cyclic antidepressants may cause sexual dysfunction, most commonly impotence in males. The SSRIs and MAOIs are more likely to cause delayed orgasm or anorgasmia in males and females. (Anecdotally, this side effect may prove a benefit in males with premature ejaculation.) Trazodone has been associated with the serious, but uncommon occurrence of priapism in males. Bupropion is the antidepressant least associated with sexual dysfunction.

11. Two cyclic compounds are problematic and are therefore not recommended by the authors. Maprotiline has produced a high incidence of seizures at dosages above 200 mg/day (and occasionally at lower doses), possibly limiting the prescription of adequate therapeutic doses. Amoxapine has neuroleptic effects making it analogous to a combination drug containing both an antipsychotic and an antidepressant, but one in which the physician has no control over the ratio. In addition, the presence of neuroleptic side effects and risks with amoxapine, such as akathisia, can needlessly complicate therapy.

12. In general, fixed combination drugs that contain a tricyclic and an antipsychotic drug (e.g., Triavil) or a tricyclic and a benzodiazepine (e.g., Limbitrol) should be avoided because they do not allow optimal titration of the component drugs for any given patient.

SELECTIVE SEROTONIN REUPTAKE INHIBITORS

The recognition that specific neuronal uptake mechanisms for serotonin were present in the CNS suggested, as early as the late 1960s, a potential target for the development of antidepressants. By the early 1970s, the technology existed for the screening of molecules that could selectively inhibit serotonin uptake. In 1972, fluoxetine was shown to produce selective inhibition of serotonin uptake in rat synaptosomes. This drug, the first of a class that includes sertraline, paroxetine, and fluvoxamine, was approved for release in the United States in December 1987. The impact of this class of drugs on the treatment of depression has been extraordinary, with more than 10 million people prescribed fluoxetine by 1994. The success of these drugs appeared to derive mainly from side effect advantages over older agents. The absence of anticholinergic, antihistaminergic, anti–alpha-adrenergic, weight gain, and cardiotoxic effects and potential for lethality in overdose generated wide patient and prescriber acceptance. This milder side effect profile made the delivery of adequate antidepressant doses available to patients for both acute and long-term treatment without need for dose titration and the endurance of persisting unpleasant or dangerous side effects. The side effects of the SSRIs may be significant, but they appear to be more tolerable than those of the older drugs. The side effects of SSRIs include initial anxiety or agitation, nausea and other gastrointestinal symptoms, and headaches in the short term and sexual dysfunction and occasionally apathy in the long term. Changes in libido or delayed ejaculation/anorgasmia may trouble as many as one-third of patients on SSRIs. While these side effects occasionally remit spontaneously, they frequently persist over time. As an alternative to switching drugs, anecdotal data suggest potential use of counteractive therapies such as yohimbine (ranging from 2.7 mg prn to 5.4 mg tid), amantadine (100–200 mg/day), cyproheptadine (4–8 mg/day, although this risks transient loss of antidepressant effect), or adjunctive low-dose bupropion, which is the one antidepressant not associated with sexual dysfunction and in some cases associated with increased libido. Very rarely SSRIs have been associated with extrapyramidal reactions.

Plasma levels of SSRIs have not been shown to correlate with efficacy and thus are not useful for therapeutic monitoring other than for compliance or to establish the safety of beginning an MAOI trial following treatment discontinuation of an SSRI.

Before Beginning SSRIs

A medical history, physical examination, and if appropriate, laboratory tests such as thyroid function tests are indicated for any patient newly diagnosed with depression. However, there are no medical tests specifically required before administering SSRIs. It is important to discuss fully with patients the common side effects that might occur; informing and reassuring the patient in this manner help the individual understand the physical symptoms that may be experienced and may enhance compliance. As with all antidepressants, it is important to stress to patients that onset of therapeutic benefit is most often delayed by several weeks and that the drugs are not effective on a prn basis.

Drug Interactions with SSRIs

The SSRIs all inhibit the hepatic cytochrome isoenzyme P450 2D6. Fluoxetine is the most potent inhibitor, followed by paroxetine, sertraline, and then fluvoxamine. However, for all of the SSRIs, vigilance is indicated concerning the possibility of increased therapeutic or toxic effects of other P450 metabolized drugs. In particular, when combining a tricyclic with an SSRI in an augmentation regimen, the tricyclic should be initiated with low doses, and plasma levels should be monitored. Also important with respect to drug interactions is the high rate of protein binding of the SSRIs, which can lead to increased therapeutic or toxic effects of other protein-bound drugs as a result of their being displaced from carrier proteins. The result is an increased amount of free and therefore active drug in the absence of a measurable increase in total plasma levels.

Use in the Elderly

Elderly patients generally tolerate the side effects of the SSRIs (and also bupropion and venlafaxine) better than they tolerate the anticholinergic and cardiovascular side effects of the tricyclic and related cyclic antidepressants. However, the elderly may have alterations in hepatic metabolic pathways, especially so-called phase I reactions, which include demethylation and hydroxylation, which are involved in the metabolism of both SSRIs and cyclic antidepressants. In addition, renal function may be decreased, and there may be increased end-organ sensitivity to the effects of antidepressant compounds. Because the elimination half-life of the SSRIs, cyclic antidepressants, and other antidepressants can be expected to be significantly greater than what it is in younger patients, accumulation of active drug will be greater and occur more slowly. Clinically this means that the elderly should be started on lower doses, that dosage increases should be slower, and that the ultimate therapeutic dose is also likely to be lower than in younger patients.

Use in Pregnancy

There is little information about the use of SSRIs in pregnancy. One prospective study of 128 pregnant women who took fluoxetine, 10–80 mg/day (mean 25.8 mg), during their first trimester did not find elevated rates of major malformations compared to matched groups of women taking tricyclics or drugs thought not to be teratogenic. There was a higher, albeit not statistically significant rate of miscarriages in the fluoxetine (13.5%) and tricyclic (12.2%) groups compared with the women exposed to known nonteratogenic drugs (6.8%). Whether this increased rate of miscarriages is biologically significant and, if so, whether it relates to the drugs or to the depressive disorder could not be determined from this study. Decisions on continuing antidepressant drugs during pregnancy must be individualized, but it must be recalled that the effects of **severe** untreated depression on maternal and fetal health may be far worse than the risks of fluoxetine or tricyclic drugs. An alternative for severe depression that appears to be safe is ECT.

Specific Drugs

Overall the SSRIs have similar side effect profiles and spectrum of efficacy. However, there are some differences meriting individual discussion.

Fluoxetine

Fluoxetine is clearly effective for major depression. There are anecdotal data that it may have particular advantages (like MAOIs) over tricyclics in treating atypical depression (discussed previously). Questions remain as to whether SSRIs are as effective as imipramine in the most serious melancholic depressions. Fluoxetine is usually begun at a dosage of 20 mg/day given in a single daily dose. It is generally given in the morning because for many patients it has a stimulatory effect; doses greater than 20 mg may be divided, with the second dose given during the afternoon. Although an antidepressant effect is usually apparent within 2–4 weeks, improvement may continue over 2 months. For that reason and because of its half-life, 2–4 days on average for fluoxetine and 7–9 days for its active metabolite norfluoxetine, it is reasonable to wait at least 4 weeks before raising the dose.

Some patients may respond to doses as low as 5 mg/day. Therefore patients with poorly tolerated side effects on 20 mg may use 10-mg capsules, mix their capsule contents in liquid, and take lower-dose aliquots, or take fluoxetine every other day, which is possible because of its long half-life. Alternatively patients may switch to another SSRI. Doses of 60–80 mg/day may be required for OCD and bulimia, but rarely appear to be required for depression. Use of the lowest effective dose will minimize side effects and therefore increase patient compliance.

The most problematic side effects of fluoxetine include agitation, neuromuscular restlessness (which may approximate neuroleptic-induced akathisia), and insomnia. These may respond to a dosage reduction or to temporary administration of a beta-adrenergic blocker or benzodiazepine. Anecdotally, clonazepam, 0.25–0.5 mg bid, has proved helpful for akathisia-like symptoms. Trazodone, 50 mg hs, has proved superior to placebo for fluoxetine- or bupropion-induced insomnia. Clonazepam, 0.5–1.0 mg hs, is an alternative. Some patients receiving both fluoxetine and trazodone complain of a loss of mental clarity. A minority of patients may develop daytime sedation from fluoxetine. Sexual dysfunction may occur in both males and females, most frequently delayed ejaculation or anorgasmia, which may lead to drug discontinuation by some patients. Unlike the cyclic antidepressants, fluoxetine does not appear to cause weight gain; some patients, especially those on higher doses, may lose weight. Fluoxetine may precipitate mania in bipolar patients. Other side effects include nausea, headache, and diarrhea.

Fluoxetine is the most potent metabolic inhibitor among the SSRIs, raising levels of many hepatically metabolized drugs including cyclic antidepressants. Fluoxetine should not be used with MAOIs; because of its long half-life, fluoxetine should be discontinued 5 weeks before starting an MAOI. Its long half-life appears to mitigate against symptoms induced by abrupt discontinuation, which have been reported with shorter-acting SSRIs. These include flulike symptoms or marked reemergence (rebound) of mood or anxiety symptoms. A major advantage of fluoxetine and other SSRIs (and also venlafaxine, nefazodone, and trazodone) is that these newer drugs are far less dangerous than cyclic antidepressants or MAOIs when taken in overdose.

Sertraline

Sertraline, like fluoxetine, is an SSRI effective for the treatment of major depression. Although less studied than fluoxetine, sertraline's spectrum of efficacy appears to be similar, with efficacy in panic disorder, social phobia, dysthymia, and atypical depressive disorders. It is effective for OCD, but some clinicians believe that it is less effective for OCD than the other SSRIs. Its efficacy and side effects in general clinical practice suggest a similar profile to other SSRIs. The half-life of sertraline is shorter than that of fluoxetine, approximately 25 hours; it has a potentially active metabolite with a half-life of 60–70 hours.

Sertraline is begun at 50 mg/day with a target dosage of at least 100 mg/day in healthy adults. The dosage range is 50–200 mg in single or divided daily doses. Compared to fluoxetine, it may have more gastrointestinal (nausea, diarrhea, and upper gastrointestinal symptoms) and less activating effects in some patients. Like fluoxetine, sertraline lacks the anticholinergic and cardiovascular side effects of cyclic antidepressants and is far less dangerous than cyclic antidepressants or MAOIs in overdose. Sertraline does not appear to cause weight gain. The most commonly reported side effects are nausea, diarrhea, agitation, and sexual dysfunction (delayed ejaculation in males or anorgasmia in males and females). Sertraline can precipitate mania. It should not be used with an MAOI. The recommended washout period before starting an MAOI is 14 days.

Paroxetine

Paroxetine was the third SSRI approved in the United States. It has proved effective in major depression in clinical trials and in general use, but like the other SSRIs, its relative effectiveness, compared with the tricyclics and MAOIs, for the most serious cases of major depression with melancholia remains a subject of debate. Its overall profile of efficacy is likely to be similar to that of fluoxetine. It has proved effective at high doses in OCD.

Paroxetine is begun at 20 mg in a single morning dose; elderly patients or those with serious hepatic or renal dysfunction should start at 10 mg daily. Patients who do not respond after 4 weeks can be increased in 10-mg increments up to a maximum of 50 mg/day or 40 mg/day in the elderly. Paroxetine is almost completely absorbed from the gastrointestinal tract and undergoes extensive first-pass metabolism in the liver. It has a half-life of 24 hours and no active metabolites and is metabolized by hepatic P450 enzymes. Thus, as with other SSRIs, elevated plasma levels have been reported in the elderly, in patients with liver disease, and in patients taking other drugs that may interfere with hepatic metabolism, such as cimetidine.

Paroxetine has a similar side effect profile to other SSRIs but has been observed in some clinical settings to be somewhat more sedating (this clinical impression has not been reported in clinical research trials). Paroxetine has also been reported to cause more constipation than other SSRIs. Other side effects are similar to those of other SSRIs, including insomnia or somnolence, nausea, "asthenia," tremor, and delayed ejaculation or anorgasmia. Unlike fluoxetine and sertraline, paroxetine is secreted at high levels in breast milk. In clinical use, paroxetine inhibits the cytochrome P450 2D6 enzymes less strongly than fluoxetine, but more than sertraline, and can be expected to cause increases in levels of drugs metabolized by these enzymes in some patients. Paroxetine may enhance the effects of anticoagulants such as warfarin, suggesting the need for close monitoring of such patients. Paroxetine should not be given with an MAOI; the washout period before starting an MAOI is 14 days.

Fluvoxamine

Although fluvoxamine has been introduced into the United States with the labeled indication of OCD only, clinical trial data and clinical experience would predict a similar spectrum of efficacy as other SSRIs including efficacy for depression. It is usually initiated in a single dose beginning with 50 mg, building up to a usual therapeutic range of 150–250 mg. It has a half-life of 15 hours. Its most common side effects are nausea, vomiting (possibly at a greater frequency than other SSRIs), headache, and insomnia or sedation. It is likely to cause sexual dysfunction similar to the other SSRIs. Although it has the least effect on hepatic cytochrome P450 2D6 enzymes of the SSRIs, it may still produce clinically significant drug interactions. It should not be used with MAOIs.

Augmentation of SSRIs

As noted previously, individuals who have not improved fully despite an adequate initial antidepressant trial may benefit from an augmentation or combination strategy. Augmentation of initial therapy with lithium, L-triiodothyronine (T_3), or another antidepressant may convert a weak or partial response to a full response without the delay required to change primary therapies altogether. To date there are more data on augmentation of tricyclic treatment than on SSRIs and other antidepressants, but some controlled data and extensive clinical experience support the use of several augmentation strategies with SSRIs.

Lithium

Lithium is combined with antidepressants in two major instances: (1) treatment of acute bipolar depression as prophylaxis against a switch into mania and (2) augmentation of an antidepressant response. Patients who are poorly responsive to SSRIs, tricyclic antidepressants, or MAOIs may benefit from addition of lithium (usually 300 mg bid–tid). Approximately half of patients may improve with a time course of several days to several weeks. (See Chap. 4 for a more extensive discussion.)

L-Triiodothyronine

A less well-established alternative to lithium augmentation is use of T_3, 25–50 μg/day. The majority of responders are said to have had normal baseline thyroid function. In some reports, responders have more often been female with prominent fatigue or psychomotor retardation. When this treatment is successful, some improvement is usually seen within 2 weeks and maximal improvement within 4 weeks.

Addition of a Second Antidepressant

The observation that some patients being transitioned from a tricyclic antidepressant to an SSRI after a poor response to the former dramatically improved on the combination led to trials of adding low doses of secondary amine tricyclics such as desipramine or nortriptyline to partial responders or nonresponders on SSRIs. Beginning with doses as low as 10 mg of the tricyclic and ranging up to 75 mg, this combination has been increasingly accepted in clinical practice as an intervention for treatment resistance or loss of benefit with SSRI therapy. Other work has suggested the possibility of a more rapid antidepressant response for some patients on a combination of fluoxetine and desipramine. Even though tricyclic doses used in this strategy are low, plasma level monitoring is recommended, since some patients will achieve substantial and possibly toxic tricyclic levels due to SSRI-induced inhibition of hepatic metabolism of the tricyclic. Less studied is the addition of other antidepressants to SSRIs or the use of other antidepressant combinations. For example, low doses of bupropion (e.g., 75–100 mg) have been reported to boost response to an SSRI, and some clinicians have employed low doses of venlafaxine instead of tricyclics in combination with an SSRI. Monoamine oxidase inhibitors should never be combined with SSRIs or with clomipramine because of the high risk of severe CNS toxicity (the so-called serotonin syndrome) and death.

Other Augmentation and Combination Strategies

Clinical practice, if not systematic study, has embraced a number of potential pharmacologic additions to ongoing SSRI therapy for incomplete or poor responders, including psychostimulants, other dopamine agonists, and buspirone. While psychostimulants may raise plasma levels of antidepressants somewhat, the improvement seen with stimulant addition is more likely due to enhancement of dopaminergic neurotransmission. Effective stimulant doses are usually determined empirically but typically are in the range of 2.5–10.0 mg bid of dextroamphetamine or 10 mg bid to 20 mg tid for methylphenidate. Stimulant abuse has not been reported with this strategy, but circumspection is in order in treating those with past history of cocaine or stimulant abuse. Adequate long-term follow-up reports are not available; however, use of stimulants is not recommended in patients who have agitation or insomnia while receiving an SSRI. Other clinical strategies based on the potential benefit of enhancing dopaminergic mechanisms have been used by some clinicians, including use of bromocriptine, pergolide, and amantadine to augment antidepressant effects, but there are no systematic data demonstrating efficacy. One controlled trial suggested a role of buspirone in accelerating or enhancing response to fluoxetine; introduced after 4 weeks of treatment in nonresponders, buspirone, up to 15 mg tid, appeared to generate an augmented response, although the possible benefit of extended treatment with the SSRI may have contributed to the outcome.

TRICYCLIC AND RELATED CYCLIC ANTIDEPRESSANTS

Chemistry

The tricyclic compounds were first developed in the 1950s. The antidepressant properties of imipramine, a structural analog of chlorpromazine, were discovered fortuitously when it was being tested as a potential antipsychotic compound. The older tricyclics (Fig. 3-2) have two benzene rings joined by a seven-member ring that contains either a nitrogen (dibenzazepines [e.g., imipramine]), only carbons (dibenzocycloheptadienes [e.g., amitriptyline]), or an oxygen (dibenzoxepines [e.g., doxepin]). A number of tricyclic and closely related tetracyclic compounds have been developed.

Pharmacology

Most of the antidepressants are available only as oral preparations, although amitriptyline, imipramine, and clomipramine are also available for parenteral use. The parenteral forms are not clearly established as more rapidly acting or more effective than oral preparations; their advantage lies in the possibility of administering them to patients who cannot or will not take oral medication. For such patients, they may provide an alternative to ECT.

Oral preparations of tricyclics and related drugs are rapidly and completely absorbed from the gastrointestinal tract; a high percentage of an oral dose is metabolized by the liver as it passes through the portal circulation (first-pass effect). The tricyclics are metabolized by the microsomal enzymes of the liver; the tertiary amines are first monodemethylated to yield compounds that are still active. Indeed, the desmethyl metabolites of amitriptyline and imipramine are nortriptyline and desipramine, respectively, and are marketed as antidepressants. Other major metabolic pathways include hydroxylation (which may yield partially active compounds) and conjugation with glucuronic acid to produce inactive compounds.

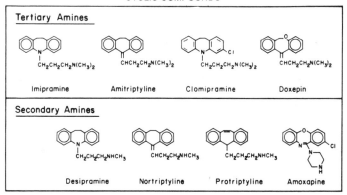

Fig. 3-2.   Chemical structures of selected antidepressants.

Tricyclic drugs are highly lipophilic, meaning the free fraction passes easily into the brain and other tissues. They are also largely bound to plasma proteins. Given their lipophilicity and protein binding, they are not removed effectively by hemodialysis in cases of overdose. The time course of metabolism and elimination is biphasic with approximately half of a dose removed over 48–72 hours and the remainder, strongly bound to tissues and plasma proteins, slowly excreted over several weeks. There is considerable variation among individuals in their metabolic rate for cyclic antidepressants based on genetic factors, age, and concomitantly taken drugs. In fact, when metabolic differences are combined with variation in the degree of protein binding, as much as a 300-fold difference in effective drug levels may be found among individuals.

Method of Use

Before Beginning Cyclic Antidepressants

A medical history and examination are indicated before beginning cyclic antidepressants, particularly to determine whether the patient has cardiac conduction system disease, which is the major medical contraindication to tricyclic use. An electrocardiogram (ECG) should be obtained for any patient with a history of cardiac symptoms or known cardiac disease; it is also reasonable as a screening test for patients over age 40. Although it appears that minor conduction system disease, such as first-degree heart block, does not increase the risk of serious sequelae from cyclic antidepressants, the presence of conduction system abnormalities favors the use of an SSRI, bupropion, or venlafaxine, as the first-choice drug. Aside from the ECG, no other tests are generally indicated in healthy adults before starting a tricyclic.

As described for the SSRIs, it is important to discuss fully with patients both common side effects of cyclic antidepressants and the expected lag period before therapeutic effects can be anticipated. Informing and reassuring the patient in this manner help the individual understand the physical symptoms that may be experienced and may enhance compliance. It should be stressed to patients that the drugs cannot be taken on an as-needed (prn) basis and are only effective if taken as prescribed. It is important for the physician to be available during the first weeks of an antidepressant trial, both to monitor the development of side effects and to help the patient differentiate effects that may be transient (e.g., dry mouth or sedation) from effects that may be more serious (e.g., postural hypotension). In this manner, both serious toxicity and noncompliance may be avoided.

Prescribing Cyclic Antidepressants

Tricyclics are started at a low dose with gradual increase until the therapeutic range is achieved. Finding the right tricyclic dose for a patient often involves a process of trial and error. The most common error leading to treatment failure is inadequate dosage. In healthy adults, the typical starting dose is 50 mg of imipramine or the equivalent. Nortriptyline is about twice as potent; thus, its starting dose is 25 mg. In some clinical situations, especially in the elderly and patients with panic disorder, it may be necessary to start with lower doses (as low as 10 mg of imipramine or the equivalent) because of intolerance to side effects.

Generally, tricyclics are administered once a day at bedtime to help with compliance and, when sedating compounds are used, to help with sleep. Divided doses are used if patients have side effects due to high peak levels. The dosage can be increased by 50 mg every 3–4 days, as side effects allow, up to a dose of 150–200 mg of imipramine or its equivalent at bedtime (see Table 3-3).

If there is no therapeutic response in 3–4 weeks, the dosage should be slowly increased, again as side effects allow. The maximum dosage of most tricyclics is the equivalent of 300 mg/day of imipramine, although rare patients who metabolize the drug rapidly may do well on higher dosages. The final dosage chosen is that at which the patient has a therapeutic response without severe side effects. Elderly patients should initiate treatment with one-third to one-half the usual adult dose with longer intervals between dosage changes.

If the patient has been on a maximal dose for 4–6 weeks without response, the drug trial should be considered a failure.

Blood Levels

There has been considerable interest in antidepressant blood levels because of the marked interindividual differences in steady state blood levels produced by any given oral dose. Many investigators have hoped to demonstrate a correlation between blood levels and therapeutic response analogous to the correlations that exist for digoxin, aminophylline, and anticonvulsants. Blood levels of tricyclic and other cyclic antidepressants are difficult to measure because the drugs circulate in very low concentrations. In general, current methods of analysis use gas chromatography, high-performance liquid chromatography, and radioimmunoassay. The literature on the relationship between antidepressant blood levels and therapeutic response often has been inconclusive or conflicting.

Of the currently available cyclic and noncyclic antidepressants, only four drugs have been studied well enough to make generalizations about the value of their blood levels in treatment of depression: imipramine, desipramine, amitriptyline, and nortriptyline. Serum levels of the other cyclic and noncyclic antidepressants have not been well enough investigated to be clinically meaningful at present except generally to confirm presence of the drug or to document extremely high serum levels.

The majority of studies of **imipramine** suggest a linear relationship between therapeutic response and blood levels of the parent compound and its desmethyl metabolite, desipramine; patients with a combined level of imipramine and desipramine greater than 225 ng/ml are believed to improve more than patients below that level. **Desipramine** given as a parent compound also appears to have a linear relationship to clinical improvement with a level greater than 125 ng/ml, producing a better response than lower levels. **Nortriptyline** levels have been the best studied of the antidepressants. They reveal a more complex pattern than imipramine or desipramine—an inverted "U" shape correlation with clinical improvement, which is sometimes referred to as a "therapeutic window." Clinical improvement correlates with levels of 50–150 ng/ml. The reason for poorer response above 150 ng/ml is not known, but it does not appear to relate to any measurable toxicity. On the other hand, the number of subjects in well-designed studies that indicate a "window" is small. Studies of **amitriptyline** levels have resulted in disagreement about the utility of levels, with linear, curvilinear, and lack of relationship reported by different investigators.

Reasons for the difficulty in unanimously establishing the utility of blood levels are unclear. It is possible that the studies reported in the literature have conflicting results because of the inclusion of mixed populations of depressives, some of whom were poor candidates for drug therapy, others of whom were appropriate for treatment, and some of whom spontaneously remitted despite subtherapeutic drug levels. In addition, the difficulty of performing tricyclic assays may have led to error in measurement of levels, especially in the early studies.

Although clinical observation and judgment are still the best method to achieve maximal therapeutic benefit without producing intolerable side effects, blood levels for imipramine, desipramine, and nortriptyline might be useful in the following limited situations:

1. To assess compliance
2. To confirm rapid metabolism, resulting in lack of both therapeutic efficacy and side effects, often due to induction of hepatic enzymes by anticonvulsants, cigarette smoking, or other agents
3. To discover slow metabolizers (i.e., patients with severe side effects at low oral doses as a result of high blood levels rather than somatization)
4. To document that a substantial level was obtained before terminating a drug trial

When used, blood levels should be drawn when the drug has achieved steady state levels (at least 5 days after a dosage change in healthy adults; longer in the elderly) and 10–14 hours after the last oral dose. One final caveat regarding tricyclic blood levels is the variability that is evident among laboratories. It is worth establishing the reliability of local laboratories if tricyclic blood levels are to be employed.

Discontinuation

As with all psychotropic drugs, it is good practice to taper cyclic antidepressants gradually rather than to discontinue them abruptly. The reasons for tapering are to prevent withdrawal symptoms (although they are relatively uncommon) and to catch reemergence of depressive symptoms so that effective doses for treatment can be rapidly restored if necessary. Withdrawal symptoms may represent cholinergic rebound, and include malaise, chills, coryza, and muscle aches. If depressive symptoms emerge during or after a drug taper, it would be reasonable to resume an effective antidepressant dosage for at least another 6 months.

Use in the Elderly

In general, the SSRIs are both safer and better tolerated than the tricyclics in the elderly. However, there have been some reports that the tricyclics may be more effective in severely ill, melancholic inpatients. Whether venlafaxine, with its tricyclic-like effect on both norepinephrine and serotonin, but without tricyclic-like anticholinergic, hypotensive, and cardiac effects, will prove to be a good alternative for melancholic elderly patients remains to be demonstrated.

As described previously, elderly patients may have slower metabolism of cyclic antidepressants, leading to greater drug accumulation and slower changes in steady state levels with dosage changes. In addition, the elderly are more sensitive to the anticholinergic effects of the cyclic antidepressants. The clinical consequence is that if a cyclic antidepressant is to be used, a less anticholinergic compound, such as desipramine, should be chosen, and compounds with very long half-lives, especially protriptyline, should be avoided. Those drugs that are used should be administered at one-third to one-half the dosage given to young patients, and the interval between dosage changes should be longer (at least 5–7 days).

In addition to these pharmacokinetic effects, the elderly are more likely to have cardiac conduction system disease that would contraindicate the use of cyclic antidepressants and are at higher risk of injury if they fall because of postural hypotension. Thus, if a tricyclic is to be used in the elderly, careful medical supervision is prudent.

Use During Pregnancy

There are limited data on the use of cyclic antidepressants during pregnancy. There have been reports of congenital malformations in association with tricyclic use, but no convincing causal association. Overall, the tricyclics may be safe, but given the lack of proven safety, the drugs should be avoided during pregnancy, unless the indications are clearly compelling. Pregnant women who are at risk for serious depression might be maintained on tricyclic therapy. This decision should always be made very carefully and with extensive discussion of the risk-benefit factors. Due to more clinical experience, older agents, such as imipramine, may be preferred to newer drugs during pregnancy.

Tricyclics appear to be secreted in breast milk. Since their effects on normal growth and development are unknown, breast-feeding should be discouraged for mothers who are on tricyclics.

Augmentation of Tricyclics

As with the SSRIs, clinicians have employed a number of augmentation or combination strategies for poor responders to a tricyclic.

Lithium

As with the SSRIs, lithium is combined with tricyclics in two major instances: (1) prophylaxis against a switch into mania in treatment of bipolar depression and (2) augmentation of tricyclic effect in treatment nonresponders. For augmentation, lithium is generally added to an established tricyclic regimen at a dosage of 300 mg bid–tid. Although initial reports found a high percentage of responders within 24–48 hours regardless of lithium level, later reports suggest a more variable response, with a delay of up to 2 weeks before improvement was evident. A small percentage relapse despite initial improvement. (See also Chap. 4).

L-Triiodothyronine

The strategy in using T_3 with tricyclics is similar to that described for its use with SSRIs. When patients have failed adequate trials of a cyclic antidepressant, 25–50 µg/day of T_3 may be added to their regimen. The mechanism of action does not appear to be an increase in tricyclic blood levels. Most responders are said to have had normal thyroid function at baseline. When this treatment is successful, some improvement is usually seen within 2 weeks and maximal improvement within 4 weeks.

Methylphenidate or Dextroamphetamine

The psychostimulants methylphenidate and dextroamphetamine have occasionally been used to augment a tricyclic regimen. For example, dosages of methylphenidate, 10 mg bid to 20 mg tid, have been used; although these doses produce a small increase in tricyclic levels, this does not seem to be the mechanism by which patients improve. This combination is successful in a small number of patients and is usually well tolerated. Patients should be monitored for onset of insomnia or agitation. This strategy is not recommended for patients with a history of psychostimulant abuse (see also Chap. 7).

Monoamine Oxidase Inhibitor

Combined tricyclic-MAOI therapy has been used in occasional cases of refractory depression. This approach has not been well studied in a controlled fashion, but there are anecdotal reports of success in cases where conventional therapies failed. Severe reactions, including fatalities, have also been reported. The most severe reactions are more likely to involve hyperthermia, seizures, and delirium than hypertensive crisis. These reactions are most frequent when a tricyclic is added to an established MAOI regimen, although they may occur at any time. If this combination is to be used, patients should be fully informed of the risks. In general, an MAOI should be slowly added to an established tricyclic regimen, or the drugs can be started at low doses together. At present, this therapy is not recommended except, perhaps, in carefully monitored inpatient settings because the risks outweigh any established benefits. Indeed, clinical experience with responders to the combination typically reveals sustained benefit when the tricyclic is withdrawn and loss of benefit when the MAOI is discontinued, suggesting that the critical agent is the MAOI.

Side Effects and Toxicity of Cyclic Antidepressants

In general the side effects of the tricyclics and related cyclic antidepressants are more difficult for patients to tolerate than the side effects of the newer drugs, such as the SSRIs, bupropion, or venlafaxine. It should be recognized, however, that many patients tolerate tricyclic drugs well, especially the less anticholinergic and less sedating compounds, such as desipramine and nortriptyline. In addition to side effects occurring with therapeutic use, another difficulty with the cyclic antidepressants (and also the MAOIs) lies in their potential for lethality in overdose.

At therapeutic levels, tricyclics may produce postural hypotension, anticholinergic (antimuscarinic) effects, and quinidine-like effects on cardiac conduction and may decrease the seizure threshold. In addition, cyclic antidepressants cause weight gain that may be significant. Should this side effect interfere with treatment, an alternative is the use of an SSRI or bupropion, neither of which is associated with weight gain. Cyclic antidepressants may cause sexual dysfunction, most frequently erectile dysfunction in males. Also, patients may experience excessive sweating, which may interfere with quality of life; if severe enough, this side effect may prompt a switch to an SSRI or bupropion (venlafaxine may also cause sweating). Most side effects of cyclic antidepressants worsen with increased doses, although some may manifest even at lower doses (e.g., dry mouth, constipation, postural hypotension). Elderly patients are generally more susceptible to these side effects. The major medical contraindication to the use of cyclic antidepressants is serious cardiac conduction disturbances.

Complaints of side effects should be taken seriously; often, however, reassurance and symptomatic treatment (e.g., stool softners for constipation, mouthwashes or sugar-free hard candies for dry mouth) are the best course. It is certainly better to help the patient tolerate side effects or to change to a different drug than to administer subtherapeutic doses. The use of subtherapeutic doses of these compounds exposes patients to side effects without providing a sufficient level of medication for treatment of the depression.

Orthostatic Hypotension

Orthostatic hypotension is the most serious common side effect of the tricyclic antidepressants and of trazodone. In the elderly, there is an increased risk of falls, with attendant increased risks of fractures and head injuries. Severe postural hypotension may limit therapy.

Postural hypotension is largely due to the alpha$_1$-adrenergic receptor antagonist properties of these drugs, although the exact mechanism is unclear. The side effect is not always dose-related, as one would expect; it often occurs at low doses and may not always worsen with higher doses. In addition, patient factors are very important—depressed patients have a higher incidence of orthostatic symptoms than normal controls on an equivalent dose of drug.

None of the cyclic antidepressants is free of this hypotensive side effect. There are conflicting reports as to whether **nortriptyline** is less likely to cause hypotension. All patients beginning tricyclics should be warned to rise slowly from recumbency or sitting positions, especially on arising in the morning. Postural blood pressures should be obtained when a patient complains of dizziness, blackouts, or falling. The newer antidepressants including SSRIs, bupropion, and venlafaxine appear to be free of hypotensive properties.

Anticholinergic Effects

Mild anticholinergic effects are common with therapeutic doses of cyclic antidepressants. These effects include dry mouth, blurred near vision, constipation, and urinary hesitancy. More severe anticholinergic effects may occur in older patients even at therapeutic dosages. These include agitation, delirium, tachycardia, urinary retention, and ileus. A common reason for the appearance of a severe anticholinergic syndrome (Table 3-5) is the concomitant use of more than one anticholinergic drug. This often is seen in clinical situations when cyclic antidepressants are used in combination with low-potency antipsychotics (especially thioridazine), antiparkinsonian drugs, antihistamines, and over-the-counter sleep medications. It is important to be aware of the possibility of precipitating an attack of narrow-angle glaucoma. Patients with open-angle glaucoma can be treated with cyclic antidepressants so long as their intraocular pressures are checked by their ophthalmologist and their glaucoma medications are adjusted as needed.

If mild-to-moderate anticholinergic symptoms interfere with treatment, bethanechol chloride, a cholinergic agent that does not cross the blood-brain barrier, may be prescribed. Effective doses

Table 3-5.   Symptoms and signs of anticholinergic toxicity

Systemic	*Neuropsychiatric*
Tachycardia	Agitation
Dilated, sluggishly reactive pupils	Motor restlessness
Blurred vision	Confusion
Warm dry skin	Disturbance of recent memory
Dry mucous membranes	Dysarthria
Fever	Myoclonus
Reduced or absent bowel sounds	Hallucinations (including visual)
Urinary retention	Delirium
	Seizures

range from 10–25 mg PO tid. For **acute urinary retention,** bethanechol chloride, 2.5–5.0 mg, may be given SQ; rarely, a urinary catheter may be temporarily required. If an anticholinergic **delirium** or severe anticholinergic syndrome is suspected, the medication should be stopped. Although the use of physostigmine can be diagnostically useful in these situations, its short half-life and toxicity limit its therapeutic use.

Cardiac Toxicity

The cardiac toxicity of tricyclic and related cyclic antidepressants may limit their clinical use (Table 3-6). The toxicity is due to the quinidine-like effects of these drugs, slowing intracardiac conduction, and to a lesser extent, to their anticholinergic effects. Patients at risk of serious cardiac toxicity are those with significant underlying conduction system disease. Except in overdose, major cardiac complications are extremely rare in patients with normal hearts (although benign ECG changes may occur).

In general, use of tricyclic and related cyclic antidepressants should be avoided in patients with bifascicular block, left bundle branch block, or a prolonged QT interval. Since the cyclic antidepressants slow intracardiac conduction, they are actually mildly antiarrhythmic, tending to decrease ventricular premature beats. Despite early reports to the contrary, cyclic antidepressants appear to have little, if any, clinically significant effects on cardiac contractility.

Sexual Dysfunction

It may be difficult to determine the true incidence of sexual dysfunction due to antidepressants because many depressed patients experience sexual dysfunction prior to initiation of treatment. Nonetheless, the incidence of sexual dysfunction with cyclic antidepressants, SSRIs, and MAOIs appears to be high in both males and females. Patients may be reticent about reporting sexual dysfunction; thus the physician should inquire about this directly at follow-up. For cyclic antidepressants, sexual dysfunction appears to be dose-related. Sexual arousal and orgasm may be impaired in both males and females. In males, erectile dysfunction is most common. The MAOIs and SSRIs also cause sexual dysfunction and therefore may not constitute a good alternative for many patients. Bupropion is the only antidepressant not associated with sexual dysfunction, and some reports indicate that it may increase libido. There are anecdotal reports that trazodone may improve sexual function in both males and females. It may rarely, however, cause medically serious priapism in males. The clinician should warn male patients on trazodone to report abnormally prolonged or painful erections immediately.

Table 3-6. Cardiac toxicity of cyclic antidepressants

Sinus tachycardia
Supraventricular tachyarrhythmias
Ventricular tachycardia and fibrillation
Prolongation of PR, QRS, and QT intervals
Bundle branch block
First-, second-, and third-degree heart block
ST- and T-wave changes

Overdoses with Tricyclic Antidepressants

Acute doses of more than 1 g of tricyclic antidepressants are usually toxic and may be fatal. Death may result from cardiac arrhythmias, hypotension, or uncontrollable seizures. Serum levels should be obtained when overdose is suspected because of both distorted information that may be given by patients and/or families and because oral bioavailability with very large doses of these compounds is poorly understood. Nonetheless, serum levels provide less specific information about the severity of the overdose than one might hope. Serum levels of greater than 1000 ng/ml represent a serious overdose, as does an increase in QRS duration or the ECG to 0.10 second or greater. However, neither of these guidelines is very exact.

In acute overdose, almost all symptoms develop within 24 hours. **Antimuscarinic effects** are prominent, including dry mucous membranes, warm dry skin, mydriasis, blurred vision, decreased bowel motility, and, often, urinary retention. **Central nervous system depression** commonly occurs, ranging from drowsiness to coma. Alternatively the patient may be agitated and delirious. The CNS depressant effects of cyclic antidepressants are potentiated by concomitantly ingested alcohol, benzodiazepines, and other sedative-hypnotics. Seizures may occur, and in severe overdoses, respiratory arrest may occur. **Cardiovascular toxicity** presents a particular danger (Table 3-6). Hypotension often occurs, even with the patient supine. A variety of arrhythmias may develop, including supraventricular tachycardia, ventricular tachycardia or fibrillation, and varying degrees of heart block, including complete heart block.

Treatment of Overdose

Basic management of overdose includes induction of emesis if the patient is alert, and intubation and gastric lavage if the patient is not. Because bowel motility may have been slowed, it is worth giving 30 g of activated charcoal with a cathartic, such as 120 ml of magnesium citrate, to decrease the absorption of residual drug.

Basic cardiorespiratory supportive care should be administered if needed. Patients with depressed respiration will require ventilatory assistance. Hypotension will require the administration of fluid (unless there is also heart failure). In refractory hypotension, or if heart failure is present, pressors such as epinephrine or phenylephrine would be the agents of choice because they counteract the anti–alpha$_1$-adrenergic effects of the antidepressant.

Any patient with arrhythmias, a QRS duration of more than 0.10 second, or a serum tricyclic level of greater than 1000 ng/ml requires continuous cardiac monitoring, preferably in an intensive care unit setting. It is sound practice to monitor levels serially and to discontinue cardiac monitoring only after serum levels are out of the toxic range and the QRS has normalized.

Sinus tachycardia usually requires no treatment. Supraventricular tachycardia contributing to myocardial ischemia or hypotension may be treated with direct-current (DC) cardioversion. Digoxin should be avoided because it might precipitate heart block, but propanolol appears to be safe in treating recurrent supraventricular tachycardia. Cardioversion is the treatment of choice for ventricular tachycardia or fibrillation. A loading dose of lidocaine and a drip of 2 mg/min may prevent recurrence. Higher doses of lidocaine may

Table 3-7.   Drug interactions with cyclic antidepressants

Worsen sedation
  Alcohol
  Antihistamines
  Antipsychotics
  Barbiturates, chloral hydrate, and other sedatives

Worsen hypotension
  Alpha methyldopa (Aldomet)
  Beta-adrenergic blockers (e.g., propranolol)
  Clonidine
  Diuretics
  Low-potency antipsychotics

Additive cardiotoxicity
  Quinidine and other class II antiarrhythmics
  Thioridazine, mesoridazine, pimozide

Additive anticholinergic toxicity
  Antihistamines (diphenhydramine and others)
  Antiparkinsonians (benztropine and others)
  Low-potency antipsychotics, especially thioridazine
  Over-the-counter sleeping medications
  Gastrointestinal antispasmodics and antidiarrheals (Lomotil and others)

Other
  Tricyclics may increase the effects of warfarin
  Tricyclics may block the effects of guanethidine

---

increase the likelihood of seizures. If lidocaine fails to prevent further arrhythmias, propranolol and bretylium are the next agents of choice. Quinidine, procainamide, and disopyramide may prolong the QRS and may precipitate heart block in tricyclic overdosed patients and should therefore be avoided. Second- and third-degree heart block can be managed by insertion of a temporary pacemaker. Physostigmine is not effective in the treatment of tricyclic-induced cardiac arrhythmias.

Central nervous system toxicity can also produce significant morbidity or death in tricyclic overdose. Generally, delirium is managed with a quiet environment and reassurance; severely agitated patients may need restraints. For patients with uncontrollable delirium that is threatening their medical condition, low doses of benzodiazepines may be effective. Because of its toxicity and short duration of action, physostigmine is not generally recommended as a therapeutic agent.

One of the most troublesome medical complications following overdose with cyclic antidepressants is seizures. First-line pharmacologic treatment for seizures induced by cyclic antidepressants is one of the benzodiazepines, diazepam or lorazepam. Diazepam is given in a dose of 5–10 mg IV at a rate of 2 mg/min. The dose may be repeated every 5–10 minutes until seizures are controlled. The risk of respiratory arrest can be minimized if intravenous benzodiazepines are given slowly, but resuscitation equipment should be available. Lorazepam is given in a dose of 1–2 mg IV over several minutes. The advantage of lorazepam is a longer biologic effect than diazepam in acute usage (hours as opposed to minutes) because of a smaller volume of distribution and perhaps a lesser tendency to respiratory depression (see Chap. 6). If a benzodiazepine fails, phenytoin should be given in a full loading dose of 15 mg/kg no more

Table 3-8. **Drugs that may affect levels of cyclic antidepressants**

Increase Levels	Decrease Levels
Acetazolamide	Alcohol (chronic use)
Antipsychotics	Barbiturates and similarly acting sedative-hypnotics
Disulfiram	Carbamazepine*
Fluoxetine* and other SSRIs	Heavy cigarette smoking
Glucocorticoids	Phenobarbital*
Methylphenidate and amphetamines	Phenytoin*
Oral contraceptives	Primidone*
Salicylates	Rifampin*
Thiazides	
Thyroid hormone	

*Major effect.

rapidly than 50 mg/min. Over-rapid administration of phenytoin causes severe hypotension.

Forced diuresis and dialysis are of no value because of protein and tissue binding of cyclic antidepressants and may exacerbate hemodynamic instability. Hemoperfusion may have a limited role in extremely severe cases, but its use must be considered experimental.

Drug Interactions

The cyclic antidepressants have a variety of important interactions that may worsen toxicity, including a variety of pharmacokinetic interactions (Tables 3-7 and 3-8).

OTHER ANTIDEPRESSANTS

Bupropion

Bupropion is a phenelthylamine compound that is effective for the treatment of depression. Bupropion is structurally related to amphetamine and the sympathomimetic diethylpropion. Thus, it is not surprising that it has been reported to possess some stimulant-like effects when used for depression.

Patients are generally begun on 100 mg bid with an increase to 100 mg tid on day 4. An antidepressant effect becomes apparent within 2–4 weeks. Patients may develop agitation, restlessness, insomnia, and anxiety soon after initiation of treatment. Should agitation occur, the dosage can be temporarily decreased, or an adjunctive benzodiazepine may be administered. For insomnia due to bupropion, as for the SSRIs, clonazepam 0.5 mg or trazodone 50 mg PO hs is usually effective. Patients who do not improve may have their dose increased to as high as 450 mg/day. Because of the risk of seizures, it is recommended that the total daily dose of bupropion be no higher than 450 mg and that no individual dose be higher than 150 mg; doses of 150 mg should be given no more frequently than q 6h. The incidence of seizures appears to be 0.4%, which is higher than other marketed antidepressants.

Bupropion lacks anticholinergic properties and does not cause postural hypotension or alter cardiac conduction in a clinically significant manner. An advantage of bupropion over the SSRIs is that it lacks significant drug interactions. Compared to other antidepressants, bupropion has the additional advantage of not being associated with sexual dysfunction; in fact, anecdotal reports impute

libido-enhancing potential to this drug. Case series and small clinical trials also suggest that bupropion may have lower risk than
other antidepressants of precipitating mania for patients with bipolar depression and for rapid-cycling bipolar II patients, in particular.
On the other hand, bupropion has been associated with switch into
mania in some patients. Bupropion is not approved for use in
patients with anorexia or bulimia because such patients were
reported to have a very high incidence of seizures in prerelease studies. Its stimulant-like appetite-suppressing properties, however,
may make it particularly useful for depressed patients who have
hyperphagia or who have excessive weight gain when treated with
standard tricyclic antidepressants.

Rare instances of ataxia, myoclonus, and dystonia have been
reported. There are reports of bupropion causing psychotic symptoms, but the incidence appears to be low.

Venlafaxine

Introduced in the United States in 1994, venlafaxine has a tricyclic-
like mechanism of action in that it inhibits the uptake of both norepinephrine and serotonin. Like the SSRIs, however, it does not
interact with other receptors associated with tricyclic side effects.
Thus venlafaxine lacks anticholinergic, antihistaminergic, and
alpha$_1$-adrenergic blocking effects. Venlafaxine is metabolized by
cytochrome P450 2D6, of which it is also a weak inhibitor. Drugs
that inhibit this enzyme may increase serum concentrations. The
half-lives of venlafaxine and its active metabolite o-desmethylven-
lafaxine are about 5 and 11 hours, respectively. The drug and this
metabolite reach steady state in plasma within 3 days in healthy
adults.

The usual dosage range is 75–225 mg given in divided doses on a
bid or tid schedule. Dosages as high as 375 mg/day have been used in
seriously ill depressed inpatients.

The side effect profile of venlafaxine is similar to that of the SSRIs.
Anxiety or nervousness may emerge or worsen on initiation of treatment. Other side effects include nausea, insomnia, sedation, dizziness, and constipation. Unlike the SSRIs, but like the tricyclics,
venlafaxine may cause sweating. At the higher doses, 5–7% of
patients may develop a modest but persisting increase in diastolic
blood pressure. Thus, baseline blood pressure screening and periodic
rechecks after upward titration of the dose should be performed.
While dose-related sexual side effects are observed with venlafaxine, early clinical reports suggest some patients with anorgasmia/
delayed ejaculation on SSRIs may not have similar problems when
switched to venlafaxine. There has been little experience with overdose, although seizure with overdose has been reported. Overall,
venlafaxine appears to be less dangerous in overdose than the tricyclics or MAOIs.

Some patients with reportedly poor responses on prior antidepressant therapies have done well in one open series with venlafaxine treatment. Venlafaxine represents an alternative to
tricyclics and will likely have a similar efficacy profile but a more
favorable acute and long-term side effect burden. Its relative disadvantage, similar to other newer drugs, is cost and lack of extensive
clinical experience. Whether its effects on blood pressure prove to be
a problem remains to be seen. Venlafaxine should be stopped 14 days
prior to initiating therapy with an MAOI.

Trazodone

Trazodone, a triazolopyridine derivative, is chemically unrelated to the tricyclics or MAOI antidepressants. Trazodone inhibits serotonin reuptake and may act as a serotonomimetic substance, possibly through its major metabolite, m-chlorophenylpiperazine (m-CPP), a postsynaptic serotonin agonist.

Trazodone is rapidly absorbed following oral administration, achieving peak levels in 1–2 hours. It has a relatively short elimination half-life of 3–9 hours and is excreted mainly in urine (75%); m-CPP has a similar pharmacokinetic profile. Despite the short half-life, once-daily dosing appears reasonable because its effectiveness is likely to reflect long-term neurochemical changes in the brain.

The therapeutic range for trazodone is 200–600 mg/day, although this has not been clearly delineated. Therapeutic blood levels have not been established. Generally, a patient can be started on 100–150 mg/day either in divided doses or in a single bedtime dose and gradually increased to 200–300 mg/day. For some patients, doses in the range of 400–600 mg may be needed. Some clinicians continue to question whether trazodone is as effective as the SSRIs, tricyclics, and MAOIs and see it as a second-line agent for major depression. Trazodone does not appear to be effective for OCD. Trazodone does appear to be useful in the treatment of SSRI-, bupropion-, and MAOI-induced insomnia in doses of 50 mg and occasionally up to 100 mg. Patients combining SSRIs or MAOIs with trazodone occasionally complain of mental clouding. Common side effects of trazodone include sedation, orthostatic hypotension, nausea, and vomiting. Side effects may be lessened if the drug is taken in divided doses and with meals. Trazodone is far less toxic than tricyclics or MAOIs in overdose.

Trazodone lacks the quinidine-like properties of the cyclic antidepressants but has been associated in rare cases with cardiac arrhythmias. Thus, trazodone should be used with caution in patients with known cardiac disease. The most common cardiovascular toxicity of trazodone is postural hypotension. This can be decreased if the drug is taken with food.

Priapism may rarely occur with trazodone, most commonly early in therapy. Males given trazodone should be instructed to report abnormally prolonged erections to their physician and/or go to an emergency room. Should priapism occur, the drug should be permanently discontinued. Trazodone may prove useful in the treatment of impotence.

Nefazodone

Nefazodone is a phenylpiperazine compound chemically similar to trazodone but with less alpha$_1$-adrenergic blocking properties and also possibly less sedation and risk of priapism. Nefazodone inhibits serotonin uptake but is also a blocker of postsynaptic 5-HT$_2$ serotonin receptors. The half-life of nefazodone is approximately 5 hours. Its most common side effects are headache, dry mouth, and nausea.

The usual starting dose is 200 mg/day given in divided doses, increased up to 300 mg in 1 week, with a range up to 600 mg if necessary. Lower starting doses are recommended in the elderly. Clinical trial data suggest that initial anxiety is less of a problem with this agent compared with the SSRIs and that sexual side effects will also be less frequent. Its safety and side effect profile appear to be quite benign, with reports of nausea, dry mouth, somnolence, dizziness, constipation, asthenia, and light-headedness most frequent in controlled trials. The drug appears to be helpful for depression-associated insomnia. Clinical experience will indicate whether it will have greater overall efficacy in addition to more tolerable side effects in comparison with trazodone.

MONOAMINE OXIDASE INHIBITORS
Iproniazid, the first of the MAOIs, was synthesized as an anti-tuberculous drug in the 1950s. It was noted clinically to have striking stimulant and antidepressant properties and was subsequently shown to be an inhibitor of the enzyme monoamine oxidase (MAO). Although its hepatotoxicity precluded its continued clinical use, other MAOIs were developed. The two MAOIs currently available in the United States for the treatment of psychiatric disorders are phenelzine and tranylcypromine.

Monoamine oxidase is found primarily on the outer membrane of mitochondria and is the enzyme primarily responsible for the intracellular catabolism of biogenic amines. In presynaptic nerve terminals, MAO metabolizes catecholamines that are found outside their storage vesicles. In the liver and gut, MAO metabolizes bioactive amines that are ingested in foods, thus serving an important protective function. It is known that MAO enzyme activity may vary markedly among individuals and appears to increase with age.

Two subtypes of MAO have been described (Table 3-9). Monoamine oxidase type A preferentially metabolizes norepinephrine and serotonin. Type B acts preferentially on phenylethylamine and benzylamine. Although selective MAOIs have been developed, the two approved for use in depression in the United States affect both the A and B types of the enzyme.

Chemistry
Phenelzine is a hydrazine derivative and an irreversible blocker of MAO, whereas tranylcypromine reversibly inhibits MAO. The other hydrazine agent, isocarboxazid, has recently been delisted by the manufacturer and is no longer commercially available. Tranylcypromine is the only available nonhydrazine MAOI antidepressant. It has structural characteristics similar to amphetamine and also has some stimulant properties (see Fig. 3-1). An additional

Table 3-9. Comparison of monoamine oxidase A and B

Type	Location	Preferred Substrates	Selective Inhibitors
A	Central nervous system; sympathetic terminals; liver; gut; skin	Norepinephrine; serotonin; dopamine; tyramine; octopamine; tryptamine	Clorgyline
B	Central nervous system; liver; platelets	Dopamine; tyramine; tryptamine; phenylethylamine; benzylamine; N-methylhistamine	Selegiline*

*Selectivity lost at higher doses ($\geq$ 10 mg/day).

MAOI, selegiline, has been approved for the treatment of Parkinson's disease. In low doses ($\leq$ 10 mg/day), as used in Parkinson's disease, it is a selective inhibitor of MAO type B and therefore does not require a tyramine-free diet. At higher doses (e.g., 30 mg/day), it may have antidepressant effects but becomes a nonselective MAOI; therefore dietary precautions must be observed.

Pharmacology

The MAOIs are well absorbed after oral administration. Parenteral forms are not available. As described, these compounds inhibit MAO in the CNS, peripheral sympathetic nervous system, and nonnervous tissues, such as liver and gut. They also partially inhibit other enzymes, but this effect probably is of little clinical consequence. With repeated dosing, maximal inhibition of MAO occurs in several days. Onset of action for antidepressant effect with MAOIs is 2–4 weeks, approximately equivalent to the latency of onset of other antidepressants. Since phenelzine irreversibly inhibits the enzyme, return of enzyme function after discontinuation may require 2 weeks (the time it takes for de novo synthesis of the enzyme). Although the bond with the MAO enzyme is not irreversible with tranylcypromine, restoration of enzyme activity may be similarly prolonged after discontinuation of the drug.

Metabolism

The metabolism of MAOIs is not well understood. There is controversy as to whether phenelzine is cleaved and acetylated in the liver. It is known that a sizable number of people are slow acetylators (a high percentage of Asians and about 50% of whites and blacks), but there is little evidence that the rate of acetylation is clinically significant for this class of drugs. Of clinical importance is the observation that metabolism of MAOIs does not seem to be affected by anticonvulsants.

MAO Levels

Although plasma levels of MAOIs are not well studied, the degree of enzyme inhibition produced by these drugs has been investigated. For phenelzine, inhibition of greater than 85% of baseline platelet MAO type B activity appears to correlate with therapeutic efficacy. Dosages greater than 45 mg/day are usually necessary to achieve this level of inhibition. This test is not useful for tranylcypromine because it maximally inhibits platelet MAO at subtherapeutic doses.

Interaction with Tyramine and Other Amines

Monoamine oxidase inhibitors inactivate intestinal and hepatic MAO (MAO type A). Thus when patients taking MAOIs ingest vasoactive amines in foods, they are not catabolized but instead enter the bloodstream and are taken up by sympathetic nerve terminals. These exogenous amines may cause release of endogenous catecholamines, which can result in a hyperadrenergic crisis with severe hypertension, hyperpyrexia, and other symptoms of sympathetic hyperactivity including tachycardia, diaphoresis, tremulousness, and cardiac arrhythmias (the clinical syndrome is described below). A number of amines (especially tyramine, but also phenylethylamine, dopamine, and others) in foods may induce these sympathomimetic crises in MAOI-treated patients. For this reason, foods containing tyramine and other vasoactive amines and sympatho-mimetic drugs should not be ingested by patients on MAOIs.

Another potentially life-threatening drug interaction involves MAOIs and agents that are serotonergic, including certain tricyclics (e.g., clomipramine), SSRIs, and buspirone. The latter agents in combination with MAOIs may result in a "serotonin syndrome," which if mild may feature tachycardia, hypertension, fever, ocular oscillations, and myoclonic jerks, but in its severe form may include severe hyperthermia, coma, convulsions, and death. There are similar life-threatening interactions with certain opioid derivatives including meperidine and dextromethorphan.

Method of Use

Generally speaking, MAOIs are at least equally effective for major depressive illness and panic disorder compared to other agents if patient selection is appropriate and adequate doses are given. Older trials in which MAOIs appeared to be less effective than tricyclics suffered from poor patient selection and, more importantly, doses of MAOIs that would now be considered subtherapeutic. More recent controlled studies (e.g., > 45 mg/day of phenelzine) have shown equivalent or greater efficacy of MAOIs compared to tricyclics. In clinical practice, MAOIs are frequently effective when all other agents have failed, and they are particularly robust therapeutic options for atypical depressives.

Nonetheless, given the complexity of their use, including dietary restrictions, MAOIs are usually reserved for patients in whom non-MAOIs have failed or have not been tolerated. In the treatment of panic anxiety complicated by polyphobic behavior, at least one study has found phenelzine to be more effective than imipramine. An MAOI may be a first-choice agent in certain patients with atypical depression or depression with panic symptoms, although given their ease of use, SSRIs are now generally preferred.

Preparing Patients for Use of MAOIs

Before beginning therapy with MAOIs, it is important to educate the patient about the risks of interactions with amine-containing foods, beverages, and medications. Patients should clearly understand the need for dietary restrictions, and it is recommended that the physician fully describe these issues before medication is prescribed. Casual prescription of MAOIs must be avoided because the risks inherent in their use require a cautious approach and a cooperative patient.

It is most useful to have a sheet of restrictions (Table 3-10) that can be given to the patient. It may be useful to enlist family support in planning meals that avoid proscribed foods. Symptoms of a hypertensive crisis should be discussed with the patient, with clear instructions to contact the treating physician immediately and/or proceed to an emergency room if symptoms occur. Patients should be questioned about compliance both with medication dosage and dietary restrictions at follow-up visits. Any signs of noncompliance should be taken seriously and corrected. If patients report "safe" transgression of dietary rules, clarification should be given that certain foods may vary in tyramine content from portion to portion; thus, successful cheating on one occasion does not rule out the possibility of a hypertensive crisis on another occasion. Given the life-threatening nature of hypertensive crises, repeated or flagrant

Table 3-10.   Sample instructions for patients taking monoamine oxidase inhibitors

1. Certain foods and beverages must be avoided:
   All **cheese** except for fresh cottage cheese or cream cheese

   Meat
   Beef liver
   Chicken liver
   Fermented sausages
      Pepperoni
      Salami
      Bologna
      Other fermented sausages
   Other cured, unrefrigerated meats

   Fish
   Caviar
   Cured, unrefrigerated fish
   Herring (dried or pickled)
   Dried fish, shrimp paste

   Vegetables
   Overripe avocados
   Fava beans
   Sauerkraut

   Fruits
   Overripe fruits, canned figs

   Other foods
   Yeast extracts (e.g., Marmite, Bovril)

   Beverages
   Chianti wine
   Beers containing yeast (unfiltered)

   Some foods and beverages should be used only in moderation:
   Chocolate
   Coffee
   Beer
   Wine

2. If you visit other physicians or dentists, inform them that you are taking an MAOI. This precaution is especially important if other medications are to be prescribed or if you are to have dental work or surgery.

3. Take no medication without a doctor's approval.

   Avoid all over-the-counter pain medications **except** plain aspirin, acetaminophen (Tylenol), and ibuprofen.

   Avoid all cold or allergy medications **except** plain chlorpheniramine (Chlor-Trimeton) or brompheniramine (Dimetane).

   Avoid all nasal decongestants and inhalers.

   Avoid all cough medications **except** plain guaifenesin elixir (plain Robitussin).

   Avoid all stimulants and diet pills.

4. Report promptly any severe headache, nausea, vomiting, chest pain, or other unusual symptoms. If your doctor is not available, go directly to an emergency room.

noncompliance with the prescribed dietary regimen should prompt the physician to consider discontinuation of the MAOI. Patients should also be made aware of proscribed medications and should be reminded to tell their other physicians and dentists that they are taking an MAOI.

In addition to dietary restriction, it is important to educate patients regarding common side effects, especially postural hypotension, insomnia, and possible sexual dysfunction. Informing patients about the latency of onset of therapeutic effects will minimize discouragement and noncompliance.

Choice of Drug

Although phenelzine has been better studied clinically, it has a greater incidence of side effects than tranylcypromine (most notably weight gain, drowsiness, anticholinergic-like effects such as dry mouth, and a greater incidence of impotence and anorgasmia). In addition, although hepatotoxicity is rare, phenelzine has a greater risk of causing serious or fatal hepatotoxicity than tranylcypromine. (It is believed that the hydrazine moiety is responsible for hepatotoxicity.)

While tranylcypromine has a lower incidence of bothersome side effects, it does cause insomnia, which may be severe. Clonazepam, 0.5 mg, or trazodone, 50 mg hs, may safely and effectively treat insomnia. Although there may be a slightly higher risk of hypertensive crisis with tranylcypromine, MAO enzyme function returns to normal more quickly when this drug is discontinued than when phenelzine is discontinued. Tranylcypromine might be the first-choice MAOI in patients who are intolerant of sedation.

Using MAOIs

Initially MAOIs are administered at low doses, with gradual increases as side effects allow. Some tolerance may develop to side effects, including postural hypotension. Phenelzine is usually started at 15 mg bid–tid (7.5–15.0 mg/day in the elderly), and tranylcypromine at 10 mg bid–tid (5–10 mg/day in the elderly). Dosages can be increased by 15 mg weekly for phenelzine and 10 mg weekly for tranylcypromine (as side effects allow) to 45–60 mg/day for phenelzine (30–60 mg/day in the elderly) and 30–40 mg/day for tranylcypromine. Dosages as high as 90 mg/day of either drug may be required, although these exceed the manufacturer's recommendations. Once depressive symptoms remit, some patients may maintain benefit on lower dosages, although in general full therapeutic doses are more protective against relapse.

Therapeutic effects often are not evident for 2–4 weeks. As with tricyclics, the aim is to achieve a therapeutic effect with the least possible toxicity. This is an empirical process that takes patience and careful dosage adjustment. Before abandoning a trial of phenelzine as a failure, some clinicians obtain a platelet MAO level. If there is inadequate suppression (85% of baseline if an initial measurement was made or 85% of normal otherwise), a higher dosage should be administered if clinically tolerated.

It is prudent to taper MAOIs over a week or so when discontinuing them; rarely, psychoses have been reported with abrupt discontinuation. When MAOIs are stopped, MAO levels do not immediately return to normal. Thus, it is prudent to wait 10 or more days before discontinuing MAOI dietary and drug restrictions after discontinuing tranylcypromine and to wait 14 days after stopping phenelzine. During changes from an MAOI to a cyclic antidepressant, similar waiting periods should be observed. Severe and even fatal interactions have been reported when tricyclics have been added to MAOIs. It is generally recommended that tricyclics be stopped for 2 weeks, fluoxetine for 5 weeks, and other SSRIs for 2 weeks before starting an MAOI.

Use in Pregnancy
There is little experience with the use of MAOIs in pregnancy. For this reason, their use should be avoided. If severe depression occurs, alternatives include SSRIs, tricyclics, and ECT.

Side Effects and Toxicity
Fear of MAOI toxicity has severely limited their use. Nonetheless, in compliant patients these drugs can be used safely and effectively.

Postural Hypotension
Postural hypotension is dose-related and may limit therapy. This side effect may be worsened markedly if patients are also receiving diuretics or antihypertensives. Patients should be advised to arise slowly from sitting positions or recumbency, especially on awakening in the morning, and to lie down if they become dizzy. Except in overdose or combined treatment with antihypertensives, episodes of hypotension almost always respond to a supine position. In the rare event of severe and unremitting hypotension, intravenous fluids are required; pressor amines should be avoided if at all possible.

Central Nervous System Side Effects
Insomnia and agitation can be troublesome side effects with tranylcypromine and rarely with phenelzine. When these occur, a trial on lower dosages should be considered. These side effects can be treated with a benzodiazepine or insomnia with trazodone. Daytime somnolence may occur with MAOIs, especially phenelzine. Patients may develop tolerance to this side effect.

Hyperadrenergic Crises
Hyperadrenergic crises are caused by ingestion of sympathomimetic drugs or pressor amines, such as tyramine, which are found in some foods and beverages. These reactions are serious and may cause stroke or myocardial infarction. All sympathomimetic drugs can lead to crises, as can L-dopa and tricyclic antidepressants (Table 3-11). Symptoms include severe headache, diaphoresis, mydriasis, neuromuscular irritability, hypertension (which may be extreme), and cardiac arrhythmias.

Patients should be advised to contact their physician and to proceed to an emergency room if any such symptoms occur. For severe reactions, **treatment** consists of blockade of alpha-adrenergic receptors with phentolamine, 5 mg IV, repeated as necessary. Phentolamine can be administered over the next 12–36 hours (0.25–0.50 mg IM q4–6h) as needed to control blood pressure. Sodium nitroprusside is extremely effective but requires continuous blood pressure monitoring for safe use. The most frequently employed strategy for mild to moderate reactions is the use of the calcium channel blocker nifedipine. In the office or emergency room, the patient is

Table 3-11.   Interactions of monoamine oxidase inhibitors with other drugs[a]

Drug	Effect
Sympathomimetics (e.g., amphetamines, dopamine, ephedrine, epinephrine [Adrenalin], isoproterenol [Isuprel], metaraminol, methylphenidate, oxymetazoline [Afrin], norepinephrine, phenylephrine [Neo-Synephrine], phenylpropanolamine, pseudoephedrine [Sudafed])	Hypertensive crisis
Meperidine (Demerol and others)	Fever, delirium, hypertension, hypotension, neuromuscular excitability, death
Oral hypoglycemics	Further lowering of serum glucose
L-Dopa	Hypertensive crisis
Tricyclic antidepressants,[b] venlafaxine[c]	Fever, seizures, delirium
SSRIs, clomipramine, tryptophan	Nausea, confusion, anxiety, shivering, hyperthermia, rigidity, diaphoresis, hyperreflexia, tachycardia, hypotension, coma, death
Bupropion	Hypertensive crisis

[a]This may include selegiline even at low doses.
[b]Tricyclics and MAOIs are occasionally used together (see text).
[c]Likely effect.

instructed to bite a nifedipine capsule and swallow the contents. Doses of 10 or 20 mg are usually initially effective and may be repeated over time to prevent or treat recurrence. Some clinicians provide patients with capsules of nifedipine in case of emergency. Beta-blockers should not be used because, as in the treatment of pheochromocytoma, their predominant clinical effect is to intensify vasoconstriction and thus worsen hypertension. After acute treatment, it is important to identify the cause of the crisis; if the cause is deliberate dietary indiscretion, continuing therapy with MAOIs should be reconsidered.

Sexual Function

Impotence, or, more frequently, delayed ejaculation in males and anorgasmia in females occurs in a substantial minority of patients. It is worth inquiring about sexual function because some patients may be embarrassed about raising the issue themselves. Cyproheptadine has been used to treat MAOI-related sexual dysfunction, but its effectiveness is questionable and it has its own side effects. Anorgasmia occasionally resolves spontaneously.

Other Side Effects

Patients have reported weight gain on all MAOIs and occasionally weight loss on tranylcypromine. Anticholinergic-like side effects occur, although they are not due to muscarinic antagonism. These side effects are less severe than those seen with tricyclics, although patients on phenelzine may experience dry mouth. Elderly patients may develop constipation or urinary retention. Alternatively, nausea and diarrhea have been reported by some patients. Sweating, flushing, or chills may also occur. Rarely, hepatitis may occur, which may be serious. Finally, some patients complain of muscle twitching or electric shock–like sensations. The latter may respond to supplementation of pyridoxine (vitamin B_6).

Overdose

Monoamine oxidase inhibitors are extremely dangerous in overdose. Because they circulate at very low concentrations in serum and are difficult to assay, there are no good data on therapeutic or toxic serum levels. Manifestations of toxicity may appear slowly, often taking up to 12 hours to appear and 24 hours to reach their peak; thus, even if patients appear clinically well in the emergency room, they should be admitted for observation after any significant overdose. After an asymptomatic period, hyperpyrexia and autonomic excitation may occur. Neuromuscular excitability may be severe enough to produce rhabdomyolysis, which may cause renal failure. This phase of excitation may be followed by CNS depression and cardiovascular collapse. Death may occur early due to seizures or arrhythmias, or later due to asystole, arrhythmias, hypotension, or renal failure. Hemolysis and a coagulopathy also may occur and contribute to morbidity and mortality.

Treatment should include gastric emptying followed by oral administration of a charcoal slurry. With the emergence of symptoms, such as delirium, hyperpyrexia, and hypertension or hypotension, meticulous supportive care is required. Central nervous system excitation can be treated with small doses of lorazepam or diazepam IV. These agents should not be used excessively, however, because they may potentiate CNS depression later. If multiple doses are to be used, lorazepam is preferred because of its shorter elimination half-life. Neuroleptics, especially low-potency agents, such as chlorpromazine, should be avoided because they can produce or worsen hypotension. Seizures may be treated with lorazepam, 1–2 mg, or diazepam, 5–10 mg, given slowly IV and repeated q10–15min as needed. Alternatively, a full loading dose of phenytoin can be administered. Severe neuromuscular irritability or rigidity may occur and may be so severe as to impair respiration because of decreased chest wall compliance. Muscular irritability and rigidity may contribute to fever, a hypermetabolic state, and rhabdomyolysis. There are several case reports of successful use of dantrolene sodium, a directly acting muscle relaxant, to treat these problems. A dosage of 2.5 mg/kg IV q6h for 24 hours was used successfully in one patient; it is prudent to continue therapy with lower doses for several days afterward. Severe hypertension may be treated with phentolamine, 5 mg IV, repeated as necessary, or with sodium nitroprusside (which requires continuous blood pressure monitoring). Ventricular arrhythmias can be safely treated with lidocaine, but bretylium should be avoided because of its adrenergic effects.

The syndrome produced by interaction of MAOIs with meperidine, dextromethorphan, and occasionally with cyclic antidepressants may be similar clinically to overdose, with similar principles of management applying.

Drug Interactions

Important drug interactions are listed in Table 3-11.

BIBLIOGRAPHY

Antidepressant Mechanism of Action

Hyman, S. E., and Nestler, E. J. *The Molecular Foundations of Psychiatry.* Washington, D.C.: American Psychiatric Association, 1993.

Indications for Antidepressants

Fluoxetine Bulimia Nervosa Collaborative Study Group. Fluoxetine in the treatment of bulimia nervosa. *Arch. Gen. Psychiatry* 49 : 139, 1992.

Goldbloom, D. S., and Olmstead, M. P. Pharmacotherapy of bulimia nervosa with fluoxetine: Assessment of clinically significant attitudinal change. *Am. J. Psychiatry* 150 : 770, 1993.

Golden, R. N., Rudarfer, M. V., Sherer, M. A., et al. Bupropion in depression: I. Biochemical effects and clinical response. *Arch. Gen. Psychiatry* 45 : 139, 1988.

Haykal, R. F., and Akiskal, H. S. Bupropion as a promising approach to rapid cycling bipolar II patients. *J. Clin. Psychiatry* 51 : 450, 1990.

Hellerstein, D. J., Yanowitch, P., Rosenthal, J., et al. A randomized double-blind study of fluoxetine versus placebo in the treatment of dysthymia. *Am. J. Psychiatry* 150 : 1169, 1993.

Jenike, M. A., Baer, L., Summergard, P., et al. Obsessive-compulsive disorder: A double-blind, placebo-controlled trial of clomipramine in 27 patients. *Am. J. Psychiatry* 146 : 1328, 1989.

Max, M. B., Lynch, S. A., Muir, J., et al. Effects of desipramine, amitriptyline, and fluoxetine on pain in diabetic neuropathy. *N. Engl. J. Med.* 326 : 1250, 1992.

Quitkin, F. M., Stewart, J. W., McGrath, P. J., et al. Phenelzine versus imipramine in treatment of probable atypical depression: Defining syndrome boundaries of selective MAOI responders. *Am. J. Psychiatry* 145 : 306, 1988.

Robinson, R. G., Kubos, K. L., Starr, L. B., et al. Mood disorders in stroke patients. *Brain* 107 : 81, 1984.

Robinson, R. G., Parikh, R. M., Lipsey, J. R., et al. Pathological laughing and crying following stroke: Validation of a measurement scale and a double-blind treatment study. *Am. J. Psychiatry* 150 : 286, 1993.

Roose, S. P., Glassman, A. H., Attia, E., and Woodring, S. Comparative efficacy of selective serotonin reuptake inhibitors and tricyclics in the treatment of melancholia. *Am. J. Psychiatry* 151 : 1735, 1994.

Spiker, D. G., Weiss, J. C., Dealy, R. S., et al. The pharmacological treatment of delusional depression. *Am. J. Psychiatry* 142 : 430, 1985.

Swedo, S. E., Leonard, H. L., Rapoport, J. L., et al. A double-blind comparison of clomipramine and desipramine in the treatment of trichotillomania (hair pulling). *N. Engl. J. Med.* 321 : 497, 1989.

Walsh, B. T., Stewart, J. W., Roose, S. P., et al. Treatment of bulimia with phenelzine. *Arch. Gen. Psychiatry* 41 : 1105, 1984.

Zisook, S., Braff, D. L., and Click, M. A. Monoamine oxidase inhibitors in the treatment of atypical depression. *J. Clin. Psychopharmacol.* 5 : 131, 1985.

Therapeutic Usage of Antidepressants

Fontaine, R., Ontiveros, H., Elie, R., et al. A double-blind comparison of nefazodone, imipramine, and placebo in major depression. *J. Clin. Psychiatry* 55 : 234, 1994.

Joffe, R. T., Singer, W., Levitt, A. J., and MacDonald, C. A placebo-controlled comparison of lithium and triiodothyronine augmentation of tricyclic antidepressants in unipolar refractory depression. *Arch. Gen. Psychiatry* 50 : 387, 1993.

Kupfer, D. J., Frank, E., Perel, J. M., et al. Five-year outcome for maintenance therapies in recurrent depression. *Arch. Gen. Psychiatry* 49 : 769, 1992.

Quitkin, F. M., Rabkin, J. G., Ross, D., and Stewart, J. W. Identification of true drug response to antidepressants. *Arch. Gen. Psychiatry* 41 : 782, 1984.

Quitkin, F. M., Stewart, J. W., McGrath, P. J., et al. Loss of drug effects during continuation therapy. *Am. J. Psychiatry* 150 : 562, 1993.

Task Force on the Use of Laboratory Tests in Psychiatry, American Psychiatric Association. Tricyclic antidepressants: Blood level measurements and clinical outcome. *Am. J. Psychiatry* 142 : 155, 1985.

Antidepressant Side Effects and Their Management

Garland, E. J., Remick, R. A., and Zis, A. P. Weight gain with antidepressants and lithium. *J. Clin. Psychopharmacol.* 8 : 323, 1988.

Johnston, A. J., Lineberry, C. G., and Ascher, J. A. A 102-center prospective study of seizure in association with bupropion. *J. Clin. Psychiatry* 52 : 450, 1991.

Marshall, J. B., and Forker, A. D. Cardiovascular effects of tricyclic antidepressant drugs: Therapeutic usage, overdose, and management of complications. *Am. Heart J.* 163 : 401, 1982.

Mitchell, J. E., and Popkin, M. K. Antidepressant drug therapy and sexual dysfunction in men: A review. *J. Clin. Psychopharmacol.* 3 : 76, 1983.

Nelson, J. C., Jatlow, P. I., and Quinlan, D. M. Subjective complaints during desipramine treatment. *Arch. Gen. Psychiatry* 41 : 55, 1984.

Nelson, J. C., Jatlow, P. I., Brock, J., et al. Major adverse reactions during desipramine treatment. *Arch. Gen. Psychiatry* 39 : 1055, 1982.

Nierenberg, A. A., Adler, L. A., Peselow, E., et al. Trazodone for antidepressant-associated insomnia. *Am. J. Psychiatry* 151 : 1069, 1994.

Rabkin, J., Quitkin, F., Harrison, W., et al. Adverse reactions to monoamine oxidase inhibitors. Part I: A comparative study. *J. Clin. Psychopharmacol.* 4 : 270, 1984.

Rabkin, J., Quitkin, F., McGrath, P., et al. Adverse reactions to monoamine oxidase inhibitors. Part I: Treatment correlates and clinical management. *J. Clin. Psychopharmacol.* 5 : 2, 1985.

Rosenstein, D. L., Nelson, C., Jacobs, S. C. Seizures associated with antidepressants: A review. *J. Clin. Psychiatry* 54 : 289, 1993.

Shulman, K. I., Walter, S. E., MacKenzie, S., and Knowles, S. Dietary restriction, tyramine, and the use of monoamine oxidase inhibitors. *J. Clin. Psychopharmacol.* 9 : 397, 1989.

Sternbach, H. The serotonin syndrome. *Am. J. Psychiatry* 148 : 705, 1991.

Verrilli, M. R., Salanga, V. D., Kozachuk, W. E., and Bennetts, M. Phenelzine toxicity responsive to dantrolene. *Neurology* 37 : 865, 1987.

Walker, P. W., Cole, J. O., Gardner, E. A., et al. Improvement in fluoxetine-associated sexual dysfunction in patients switched to bupropion. *J. Clin. Psychiatry* 54 : 459, 1993.

Antidepressant Overdose

Boehnert, M. T., and Lovejoy, F. H. Value of the QRS duration versus the serum drug level in predicting seizures and ventricular arrhythmias after an acute overdose of tricyclic antidepressants. *N. Engl. J. Med.* 313 : 474, 1985.

Knudsen, K., and Heath, A. Effects of self-poisoning with maprotiline. *Br. Med. J.* 288 : 601, 1984.

Linden, C. H., Rumack, B. H., and Strehlke, C. Monoamine oxidase inhibitor overdose. *Ann. Emerg. Med.* 13 : 1137, 1984.

Litovitz, T. L., and Troutman, W. G. Amoxapine overdosage: Seizures and fatalities. *J.A.M.A.* 250 : 1069, 1983.

Antidepressants in Pregnancy

Pastuszak, A., Schick-Boschetto, B., Zuber, C., et al. Pregnancy outcome following first-trimester exposure to fluoxetine (Prozac) *J.A.M.A.* 269 : 2246, 1993.

4

Lithium

Lithium is the oldest and best established of the mood-stabilizing agents, a group of drugs that also includes valproate and carbamazepine (see Chap. 5). Lithium is the lightest solid element in the periodic table; it is active as a psychopharmacologic agent in the form of its singly charged cation. The therapeutic value of lithium was discovered serendipitously by Cade in 1949 when he noted its calming effect on animals. He then tried it on 10 manic patients and found dramatic improvement. The therapeutic usage of lithium was thereafter rapidly explored in Australia and Europe. Its approval for use in the United States, however, was delayed until 1970 because of severe and sometimes fatal cases of lithium poisoning in the 1940s in patients who had unrestricted use of it as a salt substitute. By the time it was approved in the United States, its efficacy as a treatment for mania had been demonstrated beyond question by research in Europe.

PHARMACOLOGY

Absorption

Lithium tablets and capsules (Table 4-1) are available as the carbonate salt, which is less irritating to the gastrointestinal tract than the chloride. Each 300-mg tablet contains 8 mmol of lithium. Since lithium is a monovalent ion, 8 mmol is equal to 8 mEq. Lithium is also available as lithium citrate syrup, containing 8 mmol of lithium per 5 ml. Lithium is well absorbed after oral administration. Standard preparations produce peak serum levels in 1.5–2.0 hours; slow-release preparations that achieve peak levels in 4.0–4.5 hours also are available. No parenteral forms are available.

Blood Levels

Lithium therapy must be guided by measurement of serum levels. Serum level, not oral dose, is highly correlated with both therapeutic and toxic effects. Levels may be reported either as milliequivalents per liter (mEq/L) or millimoles per liter (mmol/L), which are equivalent since lithium ion is monovalent. Lithium levels are accurately measured by flame-photometry or atomic absorption methods that are identical to those used for sodium and potassium. Standards

Table 4-1. Available preparations of lithium

Form	Brand Name	How Supplied
Lithium carbonate	Eskalith	300-mg capsules, tablets
	Lithium carbonate	300-mg capsules, tablets
	Lithonate	300-mg capsules
	Lithotabs	300-mg tablets
Lithium carbonate, slow release	Lithobid	300-mg tablets
	Eskalith CR	450-mg tablets
Lithium citrate syrup	Cibalith-S	8 mEq/5 ml*
	Lithium citrate syrup	8 mEq/5 ml*

*8 mEq of lithium is equivalent to 300 mg of lithium carbonate.

for interpreting serum lithium levels are based on measurement 12 hours after the last oral dose (generally prior to the first morning dose). Regimens in which the entire dose is given at bedtime will produce morning levels 10–20% higher than regimens with divided dosing.

Distribution

Lithium distributes throughout total body water, although neuronal levels may be slightly lower than serum levels. There is some lag in penetration into the cerebrospinal fluid, but equilibration between blood and brain occurs within 24 hours. Like sodium, lithium circulates unbound to plasma proteins. In the elderly, there is a reduction in lean body mass (and thus total body water) of 10–15%; thus, lithium has a smaller volume of distribution in the elderly than in younger patients. This reduction, along with age-related decreases in glomerular filtration rate, contributes to the need for lower oral doses in the elderly.

Excretion

Lithium is excreted almost entirely (>95%) by the kidney. It is filtered by the glomerulus, and like sodium, it is 70–80% reabsorbed in the proximal renal tubules; lithium is also reabsorbed to a lesser extent in the loop of Henle, but unlike sodium it is not further reabsorbed in the distal tubules. Thus, its excretion is not facilitated by diuretics (such as thiazides), which act at the distal tubules. In fact, since proximal reabsorption of lithium and sodium is competitive, a deficiency of sodium, as may be produced by thiazide diuretics, dehydration, or sodium restriction, increases retention of lithium by the proximal nephron and thus increases serum lithium levels. Typically, thiazides increase lithium levels by about 30–50%, thus requiring dosage reductions in lithium if they are coadministered. On the other hand, the diuretic furosemide, which acts proximally to thiazides in the nephron (at the loop of Henle), apparently blocks lithium reabsorption to an adequate degree that it does not generally elevate serum lithium levels. Nonetheless, lithium levels must be monitored closely in any patient initiating diuretic therapy.

The renal excretion of lithium is maximal in the first few hours after peak levels are achieved and then proceeds more slowly over several days. In healthy adults, the **elimination half-life** of lithium is approximately 24 ± 8 hours. Lithium excretion is directly related to glomerular filtration rate (GFR). In the elderly, who have diminished GFR, the elimination half-life may be significantly prolonged; it may also be increased with renal dysfunction. Conversely, conditions that increase GFR, such as pregnancy, increase lithium clearance.

MECHANISM OF ACTION

Lithium has many neurobiologic effects; it is not yet certain, however, which of these effects are relevant to its therapeutic mechanism of action. Neurotransmitter receptors are proteins that span the neuronal membrane; they have extracellular ligand binding domains accessible to neurotransmitters in the synaptic space and other domains that transduce neurotransmitter binding into an intracellular effect. The reversible binding of the neurotransmitter to the receptor causes a conformational change that triggers the transmembrane signaling event. The known neurotransmitter receptors produce two different general classes of effects; they can directly control or gate the opening of an ion channel that is an intrinsic part of the receptor molecule itself, or they can act by regulating the function of a signal-transducing **G protein** that is associated with the inner surface of the membrane. The activation of G proteins initiates a complex series of biochemical actions within the cell including the regulation of certain receptor-independent ion channels and the regulation of intracellular second-messenger pathways. Many neurotransmitter receptors, including most of the receptors for monoamines (e.g., norepinephrine, serotonin, and dopamine) and all of the known neuropeptide receptors, produce their effects via G protein–linked receptors. Unlike most psychopharmacologic agents, lithium does not produce its actions within synapses but rather produces its effects intracellularly, acting directly on G proteins and second-messenger systems.

Lithium inhibits with coupling of certain neurotransmitter receptors to G proteins. It also has inhibitory effects on two second-messenger systems. Lithium inhibits receptor-mediated activation of adenylyl cyclase, the enzyme that generates the second messenger, cyclic adenosine monophosphate (cAMP). Since this effect occurs largely at lithium concentrations higher than those used clinically, it is unlikely that this is the mechanism of therapeutic action. Nonetheless, inhibition of adenylyl cyclase may contribute to some of lithium's toxic effects. Lithium may inhibit activation of adenylyl cyclase by antidiuretic hormone (ADH) and by thyroid-stimulating hormone (TSH). These actions may partly explain its tendency to cause defects in urine concentration ability and synthesis of thyroid hormones.

At concentrations achieved therapeutically, lithium acts on another second-messenger system, a pathway mediated by receptor-stimulated cleavage of a membrane phospholipid, phosphatidylinositol bisphosphate (PIP_2) (Fig. 4-1). This is currently the leading candidate mechanism of lithium action. Stimulation of certain neurotransmitter receptors (e.g., alpha$_1$-adrenergic receptors or 5-HT$_2$ serotonin receptors) leads, via G-protein activation, to the cleavage of PIP_2 by an enzyme, phospholipase C (PLC). The cleavage of PIP_2 yields two second messengers, diacylglycerol and inositol triphosphate (IP_3). IP_3 acts, in turn, to release calcium from intracellular stores. Calcium and diacylglycerol both activate protein kinases, affecting many cellular processes.

Lithium blocks the ability of neurons to restore normal levels of PIP_2 after it is hydrolyzed by PLC. All cells regenerate PIP_2 from free inositol and lipid groups. Most cells can obtain free inositol from serum; however, inositol cannot cross the blood-brain barrier. Thus unlike other organs, the brain **must** generate its own free inositol either by dephosphorylating inositol phosphates (i.e., recycling from IP_3) or by de novo synthesis from glucose-6-phosphate. Lithium inhibits the enzymes that remove the phosphate groups from inositol phosphates, thus blocking both the recycling and the de novo synthesis pathways (Fig. 4-1). The theory of lithium action is that when neurons are firing at high rates (as might occur in some cell groups during mania), those that are treated with Li$^+$ will deplete their pools of PIP_2, thus dampening their ability to respond to further stimulation by receptors that utilize this signaling pathway.

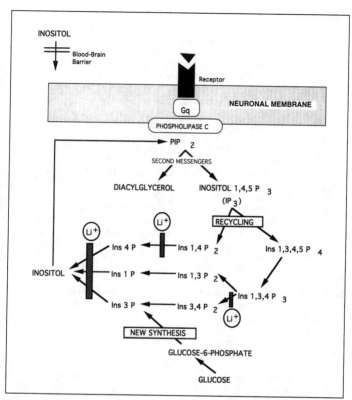

Fig. 4.1.   The effects of lithium (Li+) on the phosphatidylinositol cycle. Lithium blocks the recycling of inositol phosphates and new synthesis of inositol from glucose, thus inhibiting the ability of neurons to generate the second messengers diacylglycerol and inositol 1,4,5-triphosphate (IP₃). Gq is the signal-transducing G protein that activates this system. PIP₂ = phosphatidylinositol 4,5-bisphosphate. (Adapted from S. E. Hyman and E. J. Nestler, *The Molecular Foundations of Psychiatry*. Washington, D.C.: American Psychiatric Association, 1993. P. 141.)

INDICATIONS

Lithium has been shown to be effective in bipolar disorder, both for the treatment of acute mania and for prophylaxis against recurrences. Its usefulness in other psychiatric disorders is less well established (Table 4-2).

Bipolar Disorder

Lithium is the best studied and appears to be the most broadly effective treatment for bipolar disorder. Approximately 70% of bipolar patients gain at least moderate benefit from lithium during some stage of their treatment. For most patients, however, lithium is not, by itself, a fully adequate treatment for all phases of their illness. Lithium is most effective in the treatment of acute mania and the

Table 4-2.   Indications for lithium treatment

Effective agent of choice
  Acute mania
  Bipolar prophylaxis
Effective, other agents preferable
  Acute bipolar depression, primary treatment
Possibly effective
  Cyclothymia
  Schizophreniform disorder
  Schizoaffective disorder
  Unipolar prophylaxis (most recent episode mild)
Conflicting or preliminary evidence for effectiveness
  Aggressive behavior
  Affectively unstable personality disorders
Unproven or ineffective
  Alcohol abuse
  Anxiety
  Bulimia
  Schizophrenia

prophylaxis of manic recurrences, moderately effective in the prophylaxis of depressive recurrences, and generally inadequate as a sole acute treatment for depressive episodes. In each of these situations, lithium may be supplemented by other drugs. During acute manias, supplementation with antipsychotic drugs and benzodiazepines is often beneficial. During acute depressive episodes, supplemental use of antidepressants is most often indicated. Because of such complexities, the clinical phases of bipolar disorder are treated separately below.

Acute Mania

Many controlled studies have demonstrated that at a serum level of approximately 1 mmol/L, lithium is effective treatment for manic episodes in approximately 70–80% of cases. Lithium has also been shown to be more effective than antipsychotic drugs used as single agents in treating acute mania. Onset of improvement with lithium usually takes at least 10–14 days, and full improvement may take 4 weeks or more. When manic symptoms are not so severe as to require immediate control of abnormal behavior, lithium may be used alone. However, when mania is severe, especially in settings where hospitalization time is limited, the onset of the therapeutic response to lithium is impractically slow. Thus, early in the treatment of acute mania, antipsychotic drugs are often used as adjuncts to lithium therapy. They are effective when administered at full antipsychotic doses (e.g., 8–10 mg of haloperidol). In contrast to the benzodiazepines, which provide only sedation, the antipsychotic drugs possess true antimanic properties. Nonetheless, because of the high likelihood of undesirable side effects at higher doses of antipsychotic drugs (see Chap. 2), benzodiazepines are often used if temporary additional sedation is required during the early treatment of acute mania (e.g., lorazepam, 1–2 mg, or clonazepam, 0.5 mg, q2h prn), in addition to lithium with or without a therapeutic dose of an antipsychotic drug.

Milder cases of mania can be treated with lithium alone. However, even mild episodes that occur in the context of lithium prophylaxis generally require the temporary addition of an antipsychotic drug. If, at the time of a hypomanic or manic breakthrough, the patient's lithium level has been maintained at 0.8 mmol/L or less, the lithium dosage can be increased to achieve a level of 1.0 mmol/L (as side effects allow) and an antipsychotic drug added until the symptoms are well controlled. The treating physician must then weigh the frequency of relapses against side effects experienced by the individual patient and decide whether to attempt future prophylaxis with a higher serum level of lithium.

In treating any acutely manic patient, a low-stimulation environment should be provided. Limits should be set clearly and firmly, and provocative interactions avoided. If hospitalized patients attempt to feign compliance with medication, mouth checks and use of liquid preparations, such as lithium citrate, may be necessary. When patients refuse treatment because their judgment is impaired by mental illness, a mechanism of substituted judgment is required. Most states require evidence that there is a high risk of serious harm if the patient remains untreated and a judicial process for establishing substituted judgment.

Although antipsychotic drugs are used commonly with lithium, one still occasionally hears concern based on older reports, which suggested that the combination of lithium and neuroleptics could cause irreversible neurologic damage. While lithium and neuroleptics can interact to produce both extrapyramidal symptoms and confusion, especially in the elderly, these effects appear to be dose-related and reversible. The reported cases of severe toxicity occurred in patients on very high neuroleptic doses, with toxic lithium levels, or both. Some had symptoms indistinguishable from neuroleptic malignant syndrome. As long as rational doses are administered and patients are examined at regular intervals, antipsychotic drugs and lithium will continue to be a safe and effective combination.

Treatment-Refractory Mania

Predictors of poor response to lithium in acute mania include a prior history of poor response, rapid cycling (see below), dysphoric symptoms, mixed symptoms of depression and mania, psychiatric comorbidity (including personality disorders), and medical comorbidity. Medical illnesses may complicate attempts to achieve adequate lithium levels. For example, the presence of renal disease alters lithium excretion and therefore requires careful monitoring of both lithium levels and salt balance. The presence of sinoatrial node dysfunction raises the question of whether it is safe to use lithium in the absence of a cardiac pacemaker. The presence of even mild dementia complicates the use of lithium (as well as all other psychotropic drugs) by increasing the risk of drug-induced encephalopathy. Comorbidity of mania with either a medical disorder or a nonaffective psychiatric disorder decreases the likelihood that patients will receive adequate lithium doses or respond well if they do.

Patients who have not shown significant response to their initial mood stabilization treatment after 2–3 weeks at therapeutic levels may be considered treatment refractory. As in the case of all apparently treatment-refractory psychiatric disorders, the diagnosis should be reconsidered and the possibility of an undetected complicating medical, psychiatric, or drug abuse disorder reexamined.

Patients who do not respond to the combination of lithium and an antipsychotic drug may respond to treatment with one of the anticonvulsants, valproate or carbamazepine. Indeed some experienced clinicians now use valproate as their initial treatment for bipolar disorder. Nonetheless, given its far longer track record of safety and efficacy, lithium remains the first drug of choice for bipolar disorder in general clinical practice.

There is reasonable evidence to suggest that some patients who do not respond to lithium alone or an anticonvulsant alone respond to combination therapy with valproate and lithium or carbamazepine and lithium. Combined therapy does, however, increase the risk of central nervous system side effects, especially in elderly patients. There have also been reports of success with a valproate-carbamazepine combination in lithium-refractory or lithium-intolerant patients. Because of pharmacokinetic interactions, the dose of valproate will usually have to be increased and the dose of carbamazepine decreased if this combination is used. Anticonvulsants may also speed the metabolism of concomitantly administered antipsychotic and benzodiazepine drugs. (The use of anticonvulsants is fully described in Chap. 5). Very severe episodes of mania that do not respond satisfactorily to first-line treatments may respond to electroconvulsive therapy (ECT). Electroconvulsive therapy has the advantage of rapidity, with remission often occurring after six treatments (with treatments given 3 times weekly). Electroconvulsive therapy is not a first-line treatment, in part because the treatment of bipolar disorder requires long-term prophylaxis, which is not provided by ECT. Thus, even after successful ECT treatment, it is still necessary to find an effective prophylactic regimen. Electroconvulsive therapy is safe and effective in patients receiving lithium or antipsychotic drugs; use of valproate or carbamazepine will elevate the seizure threshold, requiring some adjustments in treatment.

Acute Bipolar Depression

Lithium is less effective in the treatment of acute depressive episodes, even in bipolar patients, than it is for acute manias and may have a longer lag time (up to 6–8 weeks) before a full response occurs. Thus, even for bipolar patients, treatment with an antidepressant—a selective serotonin reuptake inhibitor (SSRI), tricyclic antidepressant, monoamine oxidase inhibitor, bupropion, or venlafaxine (see Chap. 3)—is frequently necessary, especially if the depressive episode has occurred while the patient is on maintenance lithium. If a depression occurs in a bipolar patient who is not currently on lithium, treatment can be started with lithium alone, with lithium plus an appropriate psychotherapy, or with lithium plus an antidepressant. The choice will depend on the patient's prior history of responsiveness and the severity of the episode. Severe episodes favor initiation of combination therapy with an antidepressant because of the long lag time and lower likelihood of full response with lithium alone. When depression occurs in bipolar patients taking lithium, it should be recalled that lithium may cause hypothyroidism, which may masquerade as or exacerbate depressions.

Careful monitoring of antidepressant therapy is necessary in bipolar patients because antidepressants may precipitate a switch into mania, and concomitant therapy with lithium or an anticonvulsant is not fully protective against such switches. Although some reports have suggested that bupropion is less likely to cause a switch than other antidepressants, there are no fully convincing data to favor any antidepressant over another in the treatment of bipolar disorder. Thus issues of efficacy and side effects should be the primary factors governing the choice of antidepressants just as they do in unipolar patients (see Chap. 3). In this situation, increased vigilance for manic symptoms is indicated. Should manic symptoms emerge, the antidepressant should be discontinued and therapy continued with a mood-stabilizing agent (lithium, valproate, or carbamazepine). Antidepressant precipitated mania often continues, however, after the antidepressant is stopped, requiring institution of full antimanic treatment, which may include adjunctive use of antipsychotic or benzodiazepine drugs as well as the mood stabilizer. Despite these risks, antidepressants are often needed in the course of bipolar disorder. It is prudent, however, to withdraw them, if possible, in bipolar patients after acute depressive episodes have passed and then to maintain the patients on a mood stabilizer alone (see Chap. 3). Another reason to limit antidepressant use in bipolar patients is that all antidepressants may accelerate the rate of cycling in a minority of patients and may precipitate or worsen rapid cycling.

Mixed Episodes

When an episode is characterized by mixed symptoms of mania and depression, the episode is best treated like acute mania, that is, with a mood-stabilizing drug (lithium, valproate, or carbamazepine) or combination. As in acute mania, ECT is generally reserved for patients who are refractory to initial drug treatments and who are so severely ill that rapid treatment is required. Patients who respond to ECT will still need subsequent pharmacologic prophylaxis. In mixed episodes, as in acute mania, adjunctive antipsychotic drugs may be indicated. Benzodiazepines are the drugs of choice for adjunctive sedation. Antidepressants are to be avoided, as they are likely to worsen the overall course of the episode. Some investigators have recommended use of thyroid hormone (thyroxine [T_4] or triiodothyronine [T_3]) for refractory mixed episodes, with the goal of bringing thyroid hormone levels into the upper range of normal. This approach requires additional study.

Prophylaxis in Bipolar Disorder

Bipolar disorder must be treated with a longitudinal view of the illness, since essentially all patients will suffer recurrences. Many open and double-blind placebo-controlled studies have confirmed that lithium decreases the frequency and severity of both manic and depressive recurrences. Lithium does not, however, eliminate recurrences. Lithium may also improve minor, but troublesome subsyndromal mood swings that occur in untreated bipolar patients. Overall experience suggests that lithium is somewhat more effective in preventing manic than depressive recurrences. Episodes of mild depression are reported by many patients. Lithium appears to be less effective for patients with a history of frequent recurrences, especially if they are rapid cyclers (more than three cycles per year). Rapid withdrawal of lithium from previously stable patients appears to predispose to early manic relapses, suggestive of a rebound phenomenon (Suppes et al., 1991; see Discontinuation of Lithium Therapy, p. 109).

If the most recent episode was a mania, prophylaxis should generally be undertaken with a continuation of the mood-stabilizing drug or drugs (lithium, valproate, or carbamazepine) that were effective for that episode. Any adjunctive antipsychotic drugs used during the acute episode should be tapered and discontinued. If the most recent episode was depressive, any acutely used antidepressant should also be tapered and discontinued, if possible, and prophylaxis continued with mood stabilizers alone. There are conflicting data on optimal lithium serum levels for prophylaxis. Although effective prophylaxis has been reported with serum levels of lithium as low as 0.4 mmol/L, a randomized double-blind prospective study of 94 patients found levels of 0.8–1.0 mmol/L clearly superior to levels of 0.4–0.6 mmol/L (Gelenberg et al., 1989). Patients assigned to the lower range had a threefold higher risk of serious recurrence, predominantly mania, than those assigned to the higher range. Moreover, patients with levels in the lower range had higher rates of cycling within episodes (mania and depression within a single relapse). The main cost of higher levels is worse side effects, which affect quality of life. However, there is now a consensus that long-term treatment with standard levels does not result in renal failure or other life-threatening complications. There is an obvious trade-off—patients maintained on lower levels are more comfortable and therefore more likely to comply, but unless an adequate level is maintained, there will be less benefit, if any. It appears to be prudent to start prophylaxis with a target level of 0.8–1.0 mmol/L and to educate and reassure patients about side effects. For patients who cannot tolerate these levels, a slow decrease can be attempted. However, it is important to chart time between recurrences and severity of recurrences at each serum level to have a clear picture of each individual's dose response.

For patients who fail lithium prophylaxis after a 6- to 12-month trial, an alternative therapy should be instituted, generally valproate alone or in combination with lithium. Carbamazepine use in long-term prophylaxis is less well supported by the existing data. Intermittent addition of an antipsychotic drug is a commonly used strategy, but given the risk of tardive dyskinesia, which may be elevated in patients with mood disorders, the total lifetime use of antipsychotics should be minimized. There is some evidence to suggest that the atypical antipsychotic drug clozapine may be effective in the treatment of treatment-refractory bipolar patients alone or in combination with lithium. Although it is generally free of extrapyramidal side effects, clozapine may produce many side effects that adversely affect the quality of life, in addition to the requirement for weekly blood drawing to detect idiosyncratic granulocytopenia (see Chap. 2).

Despite the cost in side effects of prophylaxis, given morbidity and life disruption caused by manic and depressive recurrences, the question of long-term prophylaxis should be raised for every bipolar patient. In addition, it has long been observed that after the first few episodes many patients begin to have more frequent recurrences. Recently, it was observed that patients with a history of multiple (more than three) recurrences are less likely to respond to lithium prophylaxis (Gelenberg et al., 1989). It is unclear whether patients with multiple recurrences have a more severe underlying disease or whether the repeat episodes themselves produce a lasting effect on the nervous system in some patients, causing an accelerating course and lithium resistance (the "kindling" hypothesis). These observations, combined with the observation that antidepressants may also worsen the course of bipolar disorder by shortening cycle length, have led some clinicians to hypothesize that long-term lithium treatment in the range of 0.8–1.0 mmol/L and minimization of antidepressant treatment, if possible, may give a patient the best chance of a relatively benign life course with bipolar disorder. It must be emphasized that this is only a hypothesis and that long-term lithium treatment is not without its costs in terms of side effects, secondary medical problems (such as hypothyroidism), daily pill taking, and blood tests.

Some patients are resistant to the idea of long-term prophylaxis. This is particularly true in adolescent populations. In making recommendations to the patient and family, the physician should take the following into account:

1. Nature of the patient's prior episode(s), including overall severity and disruptiveness (e.g., problems with school or work, financial or legal problems)
2. Frequency and pattern of episodes (frequency often increases after the first few episodes)
3. Time course of onset of episodes (rapid onsets, which allow little time for intervention, strongly favor prophylactic treatment)
4. Patient's medical history, including need for medications that interact with lithium
5. Patient's degree of compliance
6. Patient's problems with side effects

Prophylaxis for Rapid-Cycling Bipolar Disorder

A minority of bipolar patients have more than three recurrences per year. These patients, defined as rapid cyclers, have a diminished response to lithium treatment, although lithium remains superior to placebo. Rapid cycling is more common in women. It occurs in pedigrees along with "classic" bipolar disorder, suggesting that it does not have a different genetic basis. A high percentage of patients have onset of rapid cycling while being treated with antidepressants. All classes of antidepressants and even ECT have been implicated in initiating rapid cycling in some cases. It has also been reported that thyroid abnormalities may predispose to rapid cycling, although this finding has not always been replicated.

In managing rapidly cycling patients, it is useful to graphically chart cycles and medications. Thyroid abnormalities should be vigorously sought and treated. Some clinicians would advocate an empirical trial of T_4 or T_3 therapy, to bring thyroid hormone levels into the high normal range, although this approach is not well validated. Trials of lithium should not be terminated too early, since some rapid cyclers will only begin to show improvement after a year of treatment, especially if antidepressants can be avoided. On the other hand, there is preliminary evidence that rapidly cycling patients may respond preferentially to carbamazepine or valproate (see Chap. 5). Thus, if a rapidly cycling patient has poor response to lithium despite an adequate trial, addition or substitution of carbamazepine or valproate should be considered. It is prudent to use antipsychotic drugs sparingly because of the long-term risk of tardive dyskinesia. Antidepressant drugs should be avoided if possible;

however, patients who do not respond to mood stabilizers alone should not be left untreated during serious depressive episodes. When needed, antidepressants should be used for the shortest time possible. If one antidepressant clearly shortens cycle length, an antidepressant from another chemical class should be tried. Bupropion may have some advantage over other antidepressants in this population, but this is not well established. Selective inhibitors of MAO A are also said to be advantageous in this population, but none is currently available in the United States. Electroconvulsive therapy may be the best antidepressant modality in some rapidly cycling patients.

Acute Unipolar Depression

Most studies concur that although lithium as a single agent has some antidepressant properties, it is not as effective as the SSRIs, cyclic antidepressants, MAOIs, or bupropion in the treatment of acute unipolar depression. Its major use in unipolar depression is in augmentation regimens (see also Chap. 3).

Lithium Augmentation of Antidepressants

Approximately 30% of patients with major depression do not improve substantially with their initial antidepressant treatment. Because it may take many weeks to observe improvement when changing from one antidepressant to another, a number of strategies, which include adding a second drug to the initial antidepressant, have been developed to convert refractory patients to responders. The effectiveness of adding lithium to an unsuccessful antidepressant trial has been confirmed in placebo-controlled double-blind studies, case reports, and clinical practice. Lithium augmentation can be successful with a wide range of antidepressants, including SSRIs, tricyclics, and MAOIs. Negative studies have also been reported. In addition, lithium augmentation has been reported to induce mania in a few cases. No correlation of clinical response with serum lithium level has been found.

Lithium augmentation may benefit approximately 50% of paients who receive it. Patients who are nonresponders on a fully adequate antidepressant regimen are generally started on lithium, 300 mg bid–tid. A blood level should be checked after 5–7 days or if there are severe side effects to ensure that the drug level is not in the toxic range. Patients who respond generally do so within 2–3 weeks of augmentation therapy, although some patients respond more rapidly.

Prophylaxis in Unipolar Depression

Patients with frequent or severe recurrences of unipolar depression are likely to benefit from long-term pharmacologic prophylaxis. Given the effectiveness of the antidepressants for this indication and the unproven effectiveness of lithium (despite some positive early studies), lithium will be used only very rarely for this indication except as an adjunct to antidepressant drugs.

Atypical Psychoses: Schizoaffective and Schizophreniform Disorders

As defined by DSM-IV, schizoaffective patients have prominent psychotic symptoms at times when they are free of affective symptoms, and they also have periods during which they suffer from major depressive or manic syndromes. Further research is needed to determine whether this is a valid disorder or a poor prognosis form of major affective disorder, or whether it represents a heterogeneous group of patients.

As defined by DSM-IV, schizophreniform disorder involves symptoms of schizophrenia, but of less than 6 months' duration. The onset of symptoms tends to be rapid rather than insidious, and patients may demonstrate confusion or perplexity at the height of their syndrome. Many, but not all, such patients lack the flat affect typical of schizophrenia. Schizophreniform disorder probably lacks construct validity as a psychiatric diagnosis. Instead, it may be seen to represent a heterogeneous group of patients, some with schizophrenia and others with an atypical presentation of a mood disorder.

Despite the need for further research on the classification of patients with schizoaffective and schizophreniform presentations, clinicians must still decide which patients should receive a trial of treatments for possible mood disorders (i.e., lithium, antidepressants, anticonvulsants, or ECT). Given the side effects of antipsychotic drugs and the increasing constraints on hospitalization time, it is obviously best if a diagnosis of a lithium-responsive disorder can be made early in treatment.

From the current state of knowledge, the following guidelines for the use of lithium in schizoaffective, schizophreniform, and other atypical psychotic disorders can be tentatively suggested:

1. Truly acute onset from good baseline functioning is more suggestive of a mood disorder than schizophrenia, even if abnormalities in mood are not prominent. A family history positive for mood disorder helps corroborate this diagnosis. Dysphoric mania may frequently be confused with schizophreniform disorder.
2. When patients have moderate to severe mood disturbance with neurovegetative signs during the course of a schizoaffective illness, lithium, valproate, carbamazepine, or antidepressants should be tried as appropriate. Lithium is the initial drug of choice for "schizomanic" presentations. Antidepressants are the drug of choice for "schizodepressed" presentations. These treatments may help with abnormalities of mood, sleep, and appetite, even if hallucinations, delusions, or thought disorder prove resistant.
3. The presence of paranoia as the sole or predominant psychotic symptom should raise the possibility of atypical mania or depression, especially if there is a family history positive for mood disorders or if there are neurovegetative signs.

Cyclothymia

Cyclothymia is defined as a chronic mood disturbance with periods of hypomania and depressed mood or loss of interest or pleasure; however, episodes are not severe enough to meet criteria for mania or major depression. There is often a positive family history for mood disorders in such patients. Personality disorders and drug abuse may masquerade as cyclothymia, so caution is required in making the diagnosis. Lithium is often helpful, although less clearly so than in bipolar disorder. As with rapid-cycling bipolar patients, it may be necessary to employ an extended trial of lithium ($\geq$ 1 year) to see improvement. Lithium in these patients is used in the same blood level range as in long-term treatment of bipolar patients.

Eating Disorders

There are scant data to suggest that lithium may be effective in bulimia. Given the dangers of lithium toxicity in individuals who abuse laxatives and diuretics, and the now well-established utility of the SSRIs and other antidepressant drugs as components of treatment for bulimia, lithium should be reserved only for bulimic patients who are also bipolar.

Alcohol Abuse

The use of lithium carbonate as a treatment for alcoholism has been debated for a number of years; some studies have suggested that lithium can decrease alcohol craving and alcohol "highs," but these results have not always been replicated or shown to be clinically significant. For example, one double-blind, placebo-controlled study found that alcoholics with therapeutic levels of lithium (0.7–1.2 mmol/L) had higher rates of abstinence than controls (Fawcett et al., 1987), but two other studies, including one large study of both depressed and nondepressed alcoholics, found lithium to be of no benefit over placebo (de la Fuente et al., 1989; Dorus et al., 1989). The results of these studies in combination with clinical experience suggest that lithium is not likely to be useful as a primary treatment for alcoholism. Lithium is indicated, however, if after detoxification it becomes apparent that a patient's alcohol abuse is secondary to or coexists with bipolar disorder. Because active alcohol abuse may complicate the safe use of lithium, lithium should not be prescribed prior to detoxification and initiation of psychosocial treatment for alcoholism.

Personality Disorders

The literature is quite divided on the utility of lithium or other mood stabilizers in treating **affective lability, emotional instability,** and **dyscontrol** in patients with borderline and other personality disorders. This lack of clarity occurs in clinical practice as well. A potential confounding variable in the study of personality disorders is the possibility that those individuals who responded to lithium (or antidepressants) had a comorbid mood disorder or a primary mood disorder that manifested itself as a personality disorder.

Serum lithium levels in putative positive responders have usually been reported to be in the range of 0.6–1.2 mmol/L. Although further research is needed to define lithium's usefulness, if any, in these emotionally unstable patients, lithium, carbamazepine, or valproate might be tried in those patients in whom mood swings and affective lability are prominent and disabling symptoms, so long as the mood stabilizer is not portrayed as a panacea, it is discontinued if it proves ineffective after an adequate trial (e.g., 12 weeks), and other treatment modalities continue.

Explosive and Violent Behavior

Some investigators have reported that lithium is effective in controlling episodic violence, especially in patients with antisocial personality disorder. Serum lithium levels between 0.6 and 1.3 mmol/L have reportedly been used. Although lithium's efficacy for this indication needs further research, it might be tried in violent individuals if there is a family history of mood disorders or if the patient has symptoms suggesting that violent behavior might be a manifestation of a mood disorder. Lithium's use should be presented to the patient and family as an empirical trial rather than a proven treatment.

THERAPEUTIC USE

Before Starting Lithium

Some consensus has developed on the minimum workup of patients prior to starting lithium therapy (Table 4-3). Some clinicians also obtain a pretreatment complete blood count (CBC) because lithium may cause a benign elevation of white blood cell count. Because lithium may depress sinoatrial node function, patients with sick sinus syndrome should probably be treated only if they have a cardiac pacemaker. There is no need to withhold lithium while waiting for the results of thyroid function tests, since there is no danger to the patient. If the patient proves to have a thyroid abnormality, it can be treated after lithium therapy has commenced. A pretreatment 24-hour creatinine clearance is not needed prior to beginning lithium unless the patient has known renal disease. If a lithium "test dose" is used for dosage prediction and low lithium clearance is discovered, or if the patient develops very high lithium levels on low doses when therapy begins, a creatinine clearance should then be performed. Measurement of creatinine clearance is also indicated if during the course of therapy there is a significant rise in the serum creatinine or a significant unexplained rise in lithium levels.

A variety of methods have been developed to predict individual dosage requirements using a test dose of lithium. In healthy adults, 600 mg can be given and a blood level drawn 24 hours later. The expected daily dose requirement can be read from a nomogram

Table 4-3. Summary: Method of lithium use

Before beginning lithium
   Medical history
   Physical examination
   Blood urea nitrogen, creatinine
   T_4, T_3 resin uptake, TSH
   Electrocardiogram (ECG) with rhythm strip recommended if patient is
      over age 50 or has history of cardiac disease
   CBC (optional)
   Human chorionic gonadotropin (pregnancy test), if appropriate
Initial dosing
   Usually 300 mg tid
   Lower doses in elderly or with renal disease (150–300 bid)
Blood levels
   Draw approximately 12 hours after the last oral dose
   At start of therapy, every 5 days to adjust dose
   Draw less frequently as levels stabilize
   For stable long-term patients, draw every 3–6 months
   Draw immediately if toxicity suspected
Follow-up monitoring (stable patients)
   Creatinine, TSH every 6 months
   For patients over age 40 or with cardiac disease, follow-up ECGs as
      indicated

Table 4-4. Prediction of lithium dose: Dosages required to achieve a
serum lithium level of 0.9 ± 0.3 mEq/L predicted from a lithium level
drawn 24 hours after a single dose of 600 mg

Level	Predicted Total Daily Dosage
< 0.05	3600 mg
0.05–0.09	2700 mg
0.10–0.14	1800 mg
0.15–0.19	1200 mg
0.20–0.23	900 mg
0.24–0.30	600 mg
> 0.30	Use with extreme caution

Source: Adapted from T. B. Cooper et al., *Am. J. Psychiatry* 130 : 601, 1973.

(Table 4-4). Lower test doses should be used in the elderly. This test
can be useful in identifying patients who are at the extremes of the
dosage range, including some patients with unsuspected renal failure. Since, however, optimal care requires slow dosage increases as
side effects allow, dosage prediction from a nomogram is no substitute for careful monitoring of side effects and levels.

Prior to starting lithium, patients should be told not to be discouraged if the onset of efficacy is slow and that prn doses are not helpful
and may be dangerous. They should also be instructed not to alter
their sodium intake, embark on a weight reduction diet, or take
diuretics or nonsteroidal anti-inflammatory agents without medical
supervision. This last warning is particularly important now that
ibuprofen and naproxyn are available over-the-counter.

Blood Levels

Safe and effective lithium therapy can only be monitored by serum
levels; oral dosage is not an adequate guideline. Since lithium levels
vary widely from peak to trough with most dosing schedules, it is
best to draw blood levels as close to 12 hours after the last oral dose
as possible, usually in the morning prior to the first daily dose. This
must be emphasized to patients because a misunderstanding will
result in confusing or uninterpretable levels. Regimens in which the
entire dose is given at bedtime are being used increasingly. These
will produce morning levels 10–20% higher than regimens using
divided dosing.

Since the half-life of lithium is approximately 24 hours and the
time to steady state for any drug is 4–5 half-lives, levels should be
drawn no sooner than 5 days after a change in dosage unless toxicity
is suspected. Levels drawn before equilibration is complete can be
misleading because they may still be on the rise. In the elderly and
in patients with renal disease, the half-life of elimination and hence
the time to equilibration is prolonged (often 7 days or more). If toxicity is suspected, lithium should be withheld and a level determined
immediately. Interpretation of the level requires that the time since
the last dose be taken into account.

Using Lithium

In healthy adults, the usual starting dosage is 300 mg tid, but
smaller dosages (e.g., 150 mg bid) should be used if the patient is

elderly or has renal disease. At the beginning of therapy, it is useful to draw levels every 5 days and to use these to adjust the dosage upward to the therapeutic range even if a dosage prediction
nomogram has been used.

Many side effects that occur early in therapy, such as nausea and
tremor, are due to absolute levels but may also occur at lower levels
of lithium if the levels are rising too rapidly. It is best to increase the
dosage slowly to avoid such side effects and to maximize patient
comfort and eventual compliance. If troublesome side effects emerge
at the beginning of therapy, the oral dosage should be temporarily
decreased and then slowly increased again after several days as side
effects allow. If there is pressure to obtain rapid symptom control,
temporary use of antipsychotics or benzodiazepines may be a better
choice.

Dosage Forms and Dosing Intervals

One of the major problems with long-term lithium therapy is patient
compliance. Compliance is clearly improved when dosing regimens
are simplified. Most patients tolerate lithium well on a twice daily
regimen, allowing omission of the often forgotten midday dose.
Indeed there is evidence that lithium may be best tolerated by the
kidney as a single nightly dose. Patients on a single daily dose have
less polyuria and fewer renal structural abnormalities than patients
on multiple daily doses (see Renal Effects, p. 111). The data suggest
that the kidney is able to tolerate higher peak levels reached with
single daily dosing but benefits from lower troughs. Studies are now
underway to examine the safety and effectiveness of alternate-day
dosing. From the current evidence, it would appear warranted to
treat patients with single daily doses, especially if they have compliance problems or severe polyuria. In any case, there appears to be no
reason to give lithium more frequently than twice daily unless the
patient has serious peak level side effects. Slow-release lithium may
help patients who have side effects at peak levels such as severe
tremor or nausea, but a minority of patients will only tolerate
lithium on a regimen of smaller, more frequent daily doses. The
slow-release preparations available in the United States have excel-
lent bioavailability and result in less dose fluctuation during the day
than standard lithium. Because their absorption is delayed, however, these preparations have a greater tendency to cause diarrhea
than regular lithium preparations.

Target Levels

As described previously, regimens in which the entire dose is given
at bedtime will produce morning levels 10–20% higher than regimens with divided dosing. The target levels described in this section
are based on divided dosing regimens. For **acute mania,** a therapeutic response is usually achieved at serum levels of 1.0–1.2 mmol/L.
There is no convincing justification for higher levels; levels greater
than 1.5 mmol/L are likely to be toxic. The oral dose that produces
therapeutic levels varies with the size of the patient and his or her
glomerular filtration rate. In healthy adults, the typical oral dose
to produce a level of 1.0 mmol/L is in the range of 1500 ± 300 mg,
but extreme doses range from 300–3000 mg. Some clinicians report
that early in the treatment of acute mania the oral doses needed to

produce a given level may be higher than later in treatment. The reasons for this clinical observation are unknown.

When rapid behavioral control is needed for acute mania, an antipsychotic should be started. Antipsychotic doses equivalent to haloperidol, 8–10 mg, are adequate; higher doses do not usually confer added benefit. For patients who remain hyperactive and agitated, a benzodiazepine may be temporarily added for sedation. This results in less risk of neurotoxicity than using high doses of antipsychotics. Lorazepam, 1–2 mg PO or IM q2h prn, or clonazepam, 0.5–1.0 mg PO q2h prn, is a reasonable choice. Once the acute symptoms have been controlled and the patient appears to have returned to his or her interepisode baseline, the antipsychotic drug should be slowly tapered and discontinued (so long as steady state therapeutic levels of lithium have already been achieved).

For **prophylaxis,** levels of 0.8–1.0 mmol/L have been shown to be more effective than lower blood levels, although they result in more side effects. If side effects are severe and may compromise therapy, the lowest effective serum level for that patient should be determined empirically. If a patient cannot tolerate lithium in the therapeutic range, substitution of valproate or carbamazepine should be considered.

Monitoring Long-Term Therapy

Following initiation of lithium therapy, patients should have a follow-up serum creatinine drawn, then another after reaching a therapeutic blood level. Follow-up electrocardiograms (ECGs) should be performed as clinically indicated. Lithium can be expected to cause a variety of benign changes in the ECG, including a pattern similar to that of hypokalemia. (It is important to make sure that the patient is not, in fact, hypokalemic.) Therapy should only be interrupted if a potentially dangerous arrhythmia emerges.

During long-term lithium use, serum levels can be obtained every 3 months as indicated (more frequently if toxicity is suspected or if noncompliance is a problem). Serum creatinine and TSH should be drawn every 6 months or if signs of renal or thyroid toxicity emerge. An unexplained rise in serum lithium levels requires an investigation of renal function.

Discontinuation of Lithium Therapy

Both open and controlled trials have documented that there is a substantial risk of new episodes of mania or depression following discontinuation of lithium even after years of stability on lithium. A review of existing studies found a high early risk of recurrent manias in bipolar patients following relatively abrupt lithium discontinuation, with over half of the recurrences occurring within the first 3 months after discontinuation. Depressive recurrences tended to come later. More striking, the survival time to 50% recurrence was 5 months, far shorter than during lithium treatment and even shorter than in previous untreated cycles (11.6 months) (Suppes et al., 1991). These data suggest a rebound effect with rapid discontinuation. In a prospective study, this group found that gradual (2–4 weeks) discontinuation of lithium diminished the risk of early recurrence (Faedda et al, 1993). Given these data, it would be prudent to taper lithium no more rapidly than 300 mg/month, unless side effects demand a more rapid taper.

USE IN PREGNANCY

Women with bipolar disorder may experience significant affective symptoms during pregnancy and are at elevated risk of developing postpartum manias or depressions. However, use of lithium, valproate, or carbamazepine during the first trimester of pregnancy is associated with increased risk of major birth defects. All women with bipolar disorder considering pregnancy or who become pregnant should receive counseling on the relative risks of pharmacologic treatment versus no treatment in their particular case. A contingency plan should be made (and discussed with the family) concerning a course of action should a severe episode occur, especially during the first trimester of pregnancy.

First-trimester use of lithium increases the risk of Ebstein's anomaly of the tricuspid valve. Overall, the incidence of serious congenital anomalies associated with maternal lithium use is estimated at 4–12% compared with 2–4% in comparison groups (Cohen et al., 1994). Because of the risks posed by all mood stabilizers, ECT is the treatment of choice for severe manic or depressed episodes. Alternatives that appear to be safer than lithium, valproate, or carbamazepine include high-potency antipsychotic drugs, benzodiazepines, and, for depression, imipramine.

Lithium use later in pregnancy may create complications for the mother. Regulation of the lithium level may be complicated by changes in maternal blood volume, which increases during pregnancy by 50%, and glomerular filtration rate, which increases 30–50%. At parturition there is a massive diuresis that can lead to lithium toxicity.

Lithium is secreted in breast milk at about half the serum levels in the mother. The effects of lithium on growth and development are unknown. Therefore, breast-feeding should be discouraged among mothers who must take lithium.

USE IN THE ELDERLY

Given the decrease in glomerular filtration rate and the decreased ratio of water to fat that occurs with increasing age, several precautions should be taken when using lithium in the elderly. Elderly patients should be started at lower dosages (e.g., 150–300 mg bid) depending on age and presence of renal dysfunction. Level drawing and dose changing should be slower to reflect the increased time to steady state ($\geq$ 7 days). In addition, the physician must be aware of any underlying cardiac disease. Elderly patients are often on drugs, such as diuretics and nonsteroidal anti-inflammatory agents, that may predispose to lithium toxicity. Finally, the elderly are more sensitive to the neurologic toxicity of lithium. The physician should carefully document the patient's cognitive function before beginning lithium and then monitor the patient for the emergence of subtle confusional states. Risks of producing confusional states are greater if the patient is on combined therapy with other drugs such as antidepressants, antipsychotics, anticonvulsants, and/or anticholinergics.

SIDE EFFECTS

Use of lithium is complicated by its **low therapeutic index**. At serum levels not much higher than therapeutic, significant toxicity may occur. Even at therapeutic levels, perhaps 80% of patients experience some side effects, although only 30% would be characterized as moderate or severe. Mild to moderate side effects can be bothersome enough to patients to limit therapy. The most common side effects include thirst, increased urination, tremor, and weight gain. Side effects are often a particular problem at the initiation of therapy when levels are rising or several hours after dosing when peak levels are achieved. Patients who develop bothersome side effects within several hours of a dose may do better on a slow-release preparation; alternatively, the dosage schedule can be altered so that the medication is administered in more frequent smaller doses, but multiple daily dosing makes compliance more difficult.

As serum levels rise, more serious toxic symptoms can be expected, but because patients have varying susceptibility, lithium toxicity is primarily a clinical diagnosis for which serum levels provide confirmation. In general, some toxicity is to be expected at levels above 1.5 mmol/L. Severe toxicity may manifest at levels as low as 2.0 mmol/L and is almost always evident at levels above 3.0 mmol/L. In addition to its dose-related toxicities, lithium may produce several idiosyncratic reactions, such as dermatologic reactions, which may occur at any level.

Gastrointestinal Side Effects

Patients treated with lithium may experience nausea, vomiting, anorexia, diarrhea, or abdominal pain. These symptoms are dose-related, emerging at higher serum levels or with rapidly rising serum levels at the initiation of treatment even if the actual level is not high. Thus, these symptoms are common at the start of treatment and are usually transient. If they occur with rising levels at the start of treatment, the dosage can be temporarily decreased and then increased again more slowly when the symptoms abate. Nausea may be minimized if lithium is given with meals or if slow-release preparations are used. However, slow-release preparations may result in a higher incidence of diarrhea than regular lithium. Patients who do not tolerate either preparation of the carbonate salt may have less gastrointestinal distress with lithium citrate syrup. Gastrointestinal symptoms that emerge late in treatment suggest the presence of toxic levels.

Renal Effects

Although lithium commonly causes defects in urine concentration ability, it rarely if ever causes renal failure in patients whose lithium levels are maintained in the therapeutic range. An early report of serious abnormalities, including glomerulosclerosis and interstitial fibrosis on renal biopsies of patients on long-term lithium therapy, raised the fear that long-term lithium therapy might lead to renal failure. Fortunately, careful longitudinal studies have failed to confirm this fear. For example, in a naturalistic study, 46 patients who had taken lithium for a mean of 8 years were compared with 16 patients undergoing renal biopsies for other reasons. The number of sclerotic tubules and atrophic glomeruli in the lithium-treated patients were slightly higher than those in controls, but the differences did not achieve statistical significance. However, the proportion of sclerotic glomeruli and atrophic tubules among lithium-treated patients was higher in patients who received lithium in divided daily doses than in those patients on once daily dosing (at the borderline of statistical significance). Of even more significance, patients on long-term lithium therapy do not appear to develop significant changes in glomerular function.

Polyuria

The most common renal problem due to lithium therapy is polyuria. This may be partly due to the antagonistic effect of lithium on the renal actions of ADH, leading to an inability to produce appropriately concentrated urine. However, other renal processes may contribute. Polyuria may occur in 50–70% of patients on long-term therapeutic doses of lithium; about 10% have a urine output of greater than 3 L/day, thus qualifying as having nephrogenic diabetes insipidus. Currently, lithium therapy is the most common cause of nephrogenic diabetes insipidus. Whether polyuria progresses with duration of therapy is unclear. One study of 32 patients on lithium for an average of 10 years found no interval change in polyuria in the most recent 2-year period of follow-up (Hetmar et al., 1987).

Polyuria, nocturia, and thirst can be very troublesome to patients. When severe, these symptoms may interfere with normal living habits and sleep. These symptoms may improve with dosage reduction and usually abate entirely when lithium is discontinued. A small number of patients, however, seem to have long-term (many months) or permanent urine concentrating defects that suggest structural damage to the kidney.

MANAGEMENT OF POLYURIA. For patients who are symptomatic from polyuria it should first be established that they are at the minimum effective lithium levels for them. Second, lithium can be administered as a single bedtime dose. Third, diuretics can be administered, because diuretics paradoxically decrease urine outputs in lithium-induced polyuria.

The potassium-sparing diuretic amiloride markedly decreases urine volumes without a major effect on lithium or potassium serum levels, so long as the patient has normal renal function. Amiloride is started at 5 mg bid and can be increased to as much as 10 mg bid if the effect is inadequate. Total doses above 20 mg/day do not have an added benefit. With amiloride, patients can remain on normal diets with unrestricted sodium. Nonetheless, it is prudent to monitor weekly lithium and potassium levels for several weeks after beginning amiloride to be sure that there are no changes.

Should amiloride not be tolerated, hydrochlorthiazide, 50 mg/day, can be substituted; should amiloride be tolerated but prove inadequately effective, hydrochlorthiazide, 50 mg/day, can be added. However, it must be recalled that thiazides alone or in combination with amiloride may increase lithium levels substantially. Thiazide diuretics reduce extracellular volume, leading to a compensatory increase in sodium reabsorption, thereby producing increased lithium reabsorption and elevation of lithium levels. Typically, thiazides used alone increase lithium levels by 30–50%. Thus if thiazides are used with or without amiloride, the lithium dosage should initially be halved and lithium levels monitored weekly; the needed oral dose to achieve the patient's therapeutic blood level can then be established. Thiazides have the additional problem of causing potassium depletion; even if the patient is also on amiloride, potassium levels should be monitored, initially on a weekly basis, until it is determined whether the patient is wasting potassium and needs potassium supplementation. When patients are on diuretics, it is prudent to obtain potassium levels when lithium levels are drawn.

Other Renal Problems

Rarely, patients have an **acute rise in serum creatinine** with the institution of lithium therapy, usually with a benign urinalysis (i.e., no cells or casts). Such cases are more common than is reported in the literature. These patients generally do not require a diagnostic renal biopsy. The majority have interstitial nephritis (tubulointerstitial nephropathy). In general, when the creatinine rises significantly in the context of lithium therapy, lithium should be discontinued and a 24-hour creatinine clearance performed. Of course, the physician should be sure that the problem is not due to an episode of lithium toxicity, dehydration, obstruction, or the addition of another medication. Patients who have acute interstitial nephritis will have markedly decreased creatinine clearance. Fortunately, when these changes are detected early, they are reversible with permanent discontinuation of lithium.

A small number of patients have been reported to develop **nephrotic syndrome** in association with lithium therapy (Wood et al., 1989). Nephrotic syndrome is usually reversed by discontinuation of lithium, but occasionally corticosteroids have proved necessary. Renal biopsies have revealed fusion of renal epithelial foot processes (minimal change disease). These patients should not be treated with lithium again.

Edema

A minority of patients develop intermittent **edema** of the lower extremities or face, unrelated to any changes in renal function. The edema often resolves spontaneously. If a medical etiology has been ruled out and the edema poses a problem for the individual, lithium-related edema can be treated with the diuretic spironolactone. If spironolactone is administered, lithium levels and electrolytes should be monitored (lithium levels may rise with the use of this drug).

Neurologic Side Effects

Mild neurologic side effects may occur with rising lithium levels at the start of therapy or with stable therapy, especially at times of peak levels. These complaints include lethargy, fatigue, weakness, and action tremor. The **tremor** is a 7- to 16-Hz action tremor similar to physiologic or essential tremor and unlike the pill-rolling tremor of parkinsonism. It is aggravated by anxiety and performance of fine motor movements. It may also be aggravated in some patients by concomitant administration of antidepressants. Tremor may be embarrassing for some patients and may impair normal daily activities involving delicate motor movements. Tremor can often be controlled by decreasing the lithium dosage, if possible, and decreasing or stopping caffeine intake and, if these maneuvers fail, by adding a beta-adrenergic blocker, such as propranolol. Propranolol, 10–20 mg, can be taken 30 minutes prior to an activity in which tremor will be a serious problem. For patients who require suppression of tremor all day, propranolol may be started at 10–20 mg bid with the dose titrated upward as needed. Patients who develop central nervous system side effects from propranolol may do better on the less lipophilic drug atenolol, 50 mg/day in a single daily dose. Coarsening of the tremor may be a sign of lithium toxicity.

Lithium may independently cause extrapyramidal symptoms (EPS) in a minority of patients and may worsen neuroleptic-induced EPS in some patients. The balance of the evidence suggests that lithium neither prevents nor predisposes to tardive dyskinesia. There have been case reports of lithium causing recurrence of neuroleptic malignant syndrome (NMS) when used in place of antipsychotic drugs in patients recovering from NMS. This may be due to the same mechanisms by which lithium causes EPS. Given the rarity of such reports, lithium may be used safely in patients who have recovered from NMS, but the possibility of recurrence should be kept in mind.

Several cases of **benign intracranial hypertension** (pseudotumor cerebri) occurring in association with lithium therapy have been reported. Patients presented with headache, blurred vision, and papilledema. If lithium is causally related to pseudotumor at all (perhaps by inhibiting cerebrospinal fluid reabsorption), the problem appears to be extremely rare. Therefore, screening fundoscopic examinations appear to be unnecessary. However, it would be prudent to perform a fundoscopic examination and to consider this diagnosis in patients who complain of severe headaches or new visual abnormalities while on lithium.

Lithium may produce **electroencephalographic changes** in a large fraction of patients, but only variable and minor effects on seizure threshold have been reported. Although worsening has been reported in some patients with complex partial (temporolimbic) epilepsy, many other such patients have improved behaviorally without a worsening pattern of seizures. In an open study of bipolar patients with seizure disorders (primary generalized seizures or complex partial seizures), lithium was effective in treating the mood disorder and did not increase the seizure frequency in patients with active seizures or induce seizures in patients whose seizures had remitted (Shukla et al., 1988). Pending new data, lithium should not be withheld from patients who have both mood and seizure disorders, but careful clinical monitoring is needed. Lithium does not affect serum levels of anticonvulsants.

The appearance of new neurologic symptoms during the course of therapy, even if mild, should raise the suspicion of lithium toxicity. A lithium level should be drawn and subsequent doses withheld until the question of toxicity is resolved. Patients may develop **moderately severe neurologic symptoms** at lithium levels not much higher than therapeutic. Some elderly patients or patients with brain lesions or dementia may develop such toxic symptoms even in the conventional therapeutic range. Moderate neurologic toxicity includes neuromuscular irritability, including twitching and fasciculations, EPS, ataxia, coarsening of tremor, dysarthria, incoordination, difficulty in concentrating, confusion, visual disturbance, and altered levels of consciousness. Symptoms of encephalopathy due to lithium, such as confusion or hallucinations, may be difficult to distinguish from the underlying illness, especially in patients who have a concomitant dementia. Lithium-neuroleptic combinations (commonly employed in mania) are more likely to produce EPS and encephalopathy than either drug alone.

Severe neurologic toxicity can cause ataxia, seizures, hallucinations, delirium, coma, and death. With lithium poisoning, permanent memory impairment and cerebellar ataxia may occur.

Cognitive and Psychological Side Effects

Patients on lithium may complain of dulling affect, a sense of depersonalization, a general "graying" of their mental life, or loss of creativity. Patients also may complain of memory disturbance and cognitive slowing. It has been difficult to study these complaints, some of which may reflect loss of valued hypomanias or mild depression. Schou (1984) followed artists on lithium and found that creativity increased, decreased, or was unchanged on lithium depending on the individual. Several investigators have found that subjective complaints of memory disturbance in their study population were partly explained as effects of aging and depression, although lithium could not be completely exonerated from impairing certain cognitive tasks. Joffe and associates (1988) tested attention, concentration, visuomotor function, and memory in 12 normal controls and 18 patients on lithium (serum levels 0.7–0.9 mmol/L) and on carbamazepine. The lithium and carbamazepine patients did not differ from controls. Further study with larger sample sizes is necessary to decide this issue. For the present, when patients complain of such side effects it makes sense to attempt prophylaxis with the lowest possible lithium level that affords the patient effective treatment. When patients complain of cognitive difficulty, a mental status examination should be performed and symptoms of depression should be elicited to rule out a treatable condition. In some cases, alternative therapies, such as an anticonvulsant, will be necessary.

Thyroid Side Effects

Lithium interferes with the production of thyroid hormones at multiple steps including iodine uptake, tyrosine iodination, and release of T_3 and T_4. Inhibition of the TSH-responsive adenylyl cyclase in thyroid cells may be responsible. Clinically, patients may develop goiter with or without some degree of hypothyroidism. Overall, approximately 5% of patients on long-term lithium develop hypothyroidism (compared with 0.3–1.3% in the general population, predominantly women). Perhaps 3% of patients on lithium will develop goiter. On the other hand, a much larger percentage develop increased levels of TSH. The clinical importance of this latter finding is not clear; treatment of TSH abnormalities in the absence of abnormalities in T_3 or T_4 is controversial. Patients with antithyroid antibodies prior to onset of lithium therapy appear to be at higher risk for development of hypothyroidism. The timing of onset of thyroid problems during lithium therapy is extremely variable.

Because of lithium's thyroid toxicities, it is important to perform baseline thyroid studies (TSH, T_4, and T_3 resin uptake). In follow-up, patients should be observed for development of goiter, and thyroid function tests (at least a TSH, which is the most sensitive for hypothyroidism) should be drawn every 6 months. Development of thyroid abnormalities does not necessitate a change in lithium therapy but rather treatment of the thyroid problem, usually in consultation with an endocrinologist or general internist. Should hypothyroidism or goiter develop, they can generally be treated by addition of thyroid hormone (e.g., synthetic T_4). Since hypothyroidism, including lithium-induced hypothyroidism, can present as refractory depression (Yassa et al., 1988), it is important to check thyroid function if the patient's pattern of depressive episodes changes in character or becomes treatment resistant.

Cardiac Toxicity

Many patients treated with lithium develop **ECG changes** such as T-wave flattening or inversion. These changes correlate poorly with serum levels, are reversible with discontinuation of lithium, and are almost always benign. It is important, however, that other possible causes of T-wave abnormalities, such as hypokalemia, are not ignored because the patient is on lithium.

Arrhythmias due to lithium have been described, almost always in patients with preexisting cardiac disease. Sinoatrial node dysfunction, including sinoatrial block and tachycardia, have been reported. These may present with dizziness, syncope, or palpitations or may be asymptomatic. They are reversible with discontinuation of lithium. Patients with preexisting sinoatrial node dysfunction (sick sinus syndrome) can only be safely treated if they have a cardiac pacemaker. Now that the calcium channel blocker verapamil is also occasionally used as a treatment of bipolar disorder, there is an increasing possibility that it will be used together with lithium. Cases of serious bradycardia with this combination have been reported.

Ventricular arrhythmias have also been reported, although rarely. In several case reports, patients were also receiving antipsychotic drugs. Now that it is known that some antipsychotics (e.g., thioridazine and trifluoperazine) are calcium antagonists, it is possible that the cause for the arrhythmias should be reassigned to the antipsychotic or to combined toxicity.

There is a report of increased incidence of **sudden death** in association with lithium therapy for leukopenia in cancer patients after chemotherapy (Lyman et al., 1984). Almost without exception the patients had underlying cardiac disease. It is impossible to generalize from this or other reports of sudden death in association with lithium. Indeed there are no clear guidelines for cardiac monitoring of patients on lithium. It is reasonable to question patients about cardiac symptoms or history of cardiac disease before initiating lithium therapy. Patients over age 50 or those who have a cardiac history should have a baseline ECG with follow-up ECGs as clinically indicated. If there is any question about cardiac disease, a consultation with an internist should be obtained. During follow-up visits, patients should be asked about dizziness, palpitations, or irregular heartbeats when they are asked about other possible side effects of lithium.

Dermatologic Reactions

Dermatologic reactions appear to be idiosyncratic rather than dose-related. They include acne and psoriasis (which are the most frequent), maculopapular eruptions, folliculitis, and extremely rare cases of exfoliative dermatitis. This last, a presumed hypersensitivity reaction, may be life-threatening; patients who recover should not receive lithium again.

Acne

Acneiform eruptions are probably the most common dermatologic reaction to lithium. They may prove to be a major stumbling block to acceptance of lithium by adolescents and young adults unless vigorously treated. The acne usually begins as a monomorphic eruption (all lesions in the same stage) and may occur on the face, neck, shoulders, and back. The eruptions may be new or an exacerbation of preexisting acne. The acne usually responds to vigorous treatment with standard anti-acne regimens. If the acne does not respond, a dermatologic consultation might be useful, especially if lithium refusal could result from the patient's cosmetic concerns.

Psoriasis

Lithium may cause exacerbations of preexisting psoriasis or onset of new psoriasis. Psoriasis due to lithium tends to be extremely treatment resistant but usually regresses with discontinuation of the drug. The decision to stop lithium must obviously be balanced with the risks to the patient from affective illness. The anticonvulsants do not appear to have any effects on this skin disorder. Some patients with preexisting psoriasis do not worsen on lithium, thus a history of psoriasis is not an absolute contraindication to lithium therapy, although patients with severe disease or psoriatic arthritis might be more safely treated with valproate or carbamazepine.

Other Dermatologic Reactions

Maculopapular rashes (usually pruritic) have been reported to occur occasionally early in treatment. These often regress by themselves. Asymptomatic folliculitis, which may occur as hyperkeratotic erythematous follicular papules on extensor surfaces, abdomen, and buttocks, has also been reported. It appears to pose little problem for patients and should not require changes in lithium therapy.

Hair loss is a rare side effect of lithium therapy. When hair loss occurs, it is important to check for hypothyroidism and other possible causes of alopecia.

Hematologic Effects

Lithium produces a benign, relative leukocytosis, increasing neutrophil mass without impairing function. There is no known adverse effect, and in fact leukocytosis induced by lithium has been exploited in the treatment of leukopenic patients. It is important to be aware of this effect of lithium to avoid unnecessary medical workups for elevated white blood cell counts. The total white blood cell count rarely exceeds 15,000 as a result of lithium therapy alone.

Weight Gain

A side effect that can be extremely troublesome and lead to noncompliance or lithium refusal is weight gain (Garland et al., 1988). In some studies, lithium has been associated with weight gain of more than 10 kg in 20% of patients on long-term therapy. Lithium has been reported to have insulin-like effects on carbohydrate metabolism. Antipsychotic drugs and cyclic antidepressants may also cause obesity (a hypothalamic mechanism has been the hypothesized cause for this). Patients who are polyuric should be advised not to replace their fluid losses with high-calorie beverages such as beer or sugary sodas. Some will benefit from dietary consultation. For some patients who have developed severe obesity, substitution of another drug for lithium might be considered.

Calcium Metabolism

Anecdotal reports and several small studies have associated lithium therapy with mild elevations in calcium and parathyroid hormone. These elevations appear to be rarely, if ever, clinically significant. However, since alterations in calcium level are associated with neuropsychiatric symptoms, a serum calcium might be obtained if there is a change in a patient's pattern of symptoms, especially depressive symptoms.

EVALUATION AND TREATMENT OF LITHIUM TOXICITY DUE TO ELEVATED LEVELS

For **mild toxicity,** lithium should be withheld until levels return to the patient's usual therapeutic range. If an obvious cause for the change in level cannot be found, a renal workup should be undertaken, including urinalysis and creatinine clearance.

For **moderate to severe lithium toxicity,** the patient is best admitted to a hospital. Adequate sodium should be given, and lithium levels should be checked several times a day to make sure that they are decreasing. If the patient does not have congestive heart failure or renal failure, intravenous administration of normal saline at a rate of 150–200 ml/hr is often effective in reducing lithium levels rapidly; this is safe as long as urine output is adequate.

Acute Lithium Intoxication

Acute lithium intoxication, manifest by a severe clinical syndrome or levels above 3.0 mmol/L, is a medical emergency. Because the severity and reversibility of toxic symptoms are related both to the serum level and to the duration of high levels, rapid aggressive treatment is necessary even if the patient appears clinically well. Indeed, early in lithium poisoning the patient's symptoms may be relatively mild despite high levels, giving the physician a false sense of security. Symptoms of serious intoxication include both systemic and neurologic symptoms, including nausea, vomiting, diarrhea, renal failure, neuromuscular irritability or flaccidity, ataxia, dysarthria, coarse tremor, confusion, delirium, hallucinations, seizures, and stupor. Protracted coma and glucose intolerance have been reported. Lithium poisoning may also cause death. Survivors of serious toxicity may suffer permanent cerebellar ataxia and severe permanent anterograde amnesia.

In treating acute lithium intoxication, the therapeutic goal is to remove lithium from the body as rapidly as possible. It is important to obtain a toxic screen to know what other agents the patient has ingested, especially if the case appears to be an intentional overdose. If the patient is stuporous or comatose, protection of the airway, with intubation if necessary, and cardiorespiratory support should be the first priority. In overdose cases in which the drug was taken less than 4 hours prior to treatment, induction of vomiting in alert patients or gastric lavage in comatose patients will help diminish the risk of worsening toxicity. Since lithium levels are often high in gastric secretions, continuous gastric aspiration can be helpful.

Despite the fact that most reports of lithium intoxication are either anecdotal or retrospective, there seems to be strong evidence that management should be aggressive. If lithium levels are less than 3 mmol/L and signs of intoxication are mild, fluid and electrolyte abnormalities should be corrected and normal saline may be administered at a rate of 150–200 ml/hr, as long as urine output is adequate. If the lithium level is greater than 3 mmol/L and signs of toxicity are severe, or if there is poor urine output or renal failure, prompt institution of dialysis is indicated. If the lithium level is above 4 mmol/L and does not respond within a few hours to saline diuresis at a rate of 250 ml/hr, dialysis is indicated regardless of the patient's clinical appearance. Hemodialysis is most effective, but where unavailable, peritoneal dialysis may be used. Lithium will reequilibrate from the tissues after a dialysis treatment, so frequent monitoring of the lithium level is important. A reasonable end point is a lithium level of 1.0 mmol/L or less 6 hours after a dialysis treatment.

Causes of Intoxication

Although overdosage is an important cause of toxic serum levels, the most common cause of toxicity among compliant patients is an **alteration in sodium balance.** Any condition that leads to sodium depletion will elevate lithium levels; thus dehydration, changes in dietary habits (either with sodium restriction or overall weight reduction diets), or the administration of sodium-wasting diuretics will cause elevations in lithium levels. There has been concern that heavy exercise or fever, both of which produce sweating, could result in lithium toxicity. However, it appears that sweat contains enough lithium that heavy perspiration does not elevate lithium levels. Other renal causes of lithium retention include many nonsteroidal anti-inflammatory agents (not aspirin, however) in susceptible individuals, intrinsic renal disease, and systemic diseases (e.g., congestive heart failure or cirrhosis) that decrease renal blood flow.

DRUG INTERACTIONS

Alcohol and other central nervous system depressants, including prescribed psychotropic drugs and antihypertensive agents, may interact with lithium to produce sedation or confusional states. Nonsteroidal anti-inflammatory agents and thiazide diuretics may increase lithium levels with resultant intoxication (Table 4-5). Metronidazole has been reported to cause serious renal toxicity when used in combination with lithium.

Table 4-5.   Pharmacokinetic interactions with lithium

Interactions that Raise Lithium Levels	Interactions that Lower Lithium Levels
Diuretics	Acetazolamide
Thiazides	Theophylline, aminophylline
Ethacrynic acid	Caffeine (mild effect)
Spironolactone	Osmotic diuretics
Triamterene	
Nonsteroidal anti-inflammatory agents	
Antibiotics	
Metronidazole (Flagyl)	
Tetracyclines	
Angiotensin-converting enzyme inhibitors	

120 Ch. 4 Lithium

BIBLIOGRAPHY

Pharmacology

Hardy, B. G., Shulman, K. I., Mackenzie, S. E., et al. Pharmacokinetics of lithium in the elderly. *J. Clin. Psychopharmacol.* 7 : 153, 1987.

Vitiello, B., Behar, D., Malone, R., et al. Pharmacokinetics of lithium carbonate in children. *J. Clin. Psychopharmacol.* 8 : 355, 1988.

Mechanism of Action

Baraban, J. M., Worley, P. F., and Snyder, S. H. Second-messenger systems and psychoactive drug action: Focus on the phosphoinositide system and lithium. *Am. J. Psychiatry* 146 : 1251, 1989.

Berridge, M. J., Downes, C. P., and Hanley, M. R. Neural and developmental actions of lithium: A unifying hypothesis. *Cell* 59 : 411, 1989.

Indications

Mood Disorders

Black, D. W., Winokur, G., Bell, S., et al. Complicated mania. *Arch. Gen. Psychiatry* 45 : 232, 1988.

Faedda, G. L., Tondo, L., Baldessarini, R. J., et al. Outcome after rapid vs. gradual discontinuation of lithium treatment in bipolar patients. *Arch. Gen. Psychiatry* 50 : 448, 1993.

Gelenberg, A. J., Kane, J. M., Keller, M. B., et al. Comparison of standard and low serum levels of lithium for maintenance treatment of bipolar disorder. *N. Engl. J. Med.* 321 : 1489, 1989.

Prien, R. F., Kupfer, D. J., Mansky, P. A., et al. Drug therapy in the prevention of recurrences in unipolar and bipolar affective disorders. *Arch. Gen. Psychiatry* 41 : 1096, 1984.

Shapiro, D. R., Quitkin, F. M., and Fleiss, J. L. Response to maintenance therapy in bipolar illness: Effect of an index episode. *Arch. Gen. Psychiatry* 46 : 401, 1989.

Small, J. G., Klapper, M. H., Kellams, J. J., et al. Electroconvulsive treatment compared with lithium in the management of manic states. *Arch. Gen. Psychiatry* 45 : 727, 1988.

Suppes, T., Baldessarini, R. J., Faedda, G. L., and Tohen, M. Risk of recurrence following discontinuation of lithium treatment in bipolar disorder. *Arch. Gen. Psychiatry* 48 : 1082, 1991.

Varanka, T. M., Weller, R. A., Weller, E. B., and Fristad, M. A. Lithium treatment of manic episodes with psychotic features in prepubertal children. *Am. J. Psychiatry* 145 : 1557, 1988.

Lithium Augmentation of Antidepressants

de Montigny, C., Cournoyer, G., Morisette, R., et al. Lithium carbonate addition in tricyclic antidepressant-resistant depression: Correlations with the neurobiological actions of tricyclic antidepressant drugs and lithium ion on the serotonin system. *Arch. Gen. Psychiatry* 40 : 1327, 1983.

Garbutt, J. C., Mayo, J. P., Jr., Gillette, G. M., et al. Lithium potentiation of tricyclic antidepressants following lack of T_3 potentiation. *Am. J. Psychiatry* 143 : 1038, 1986.

Pope, H. G., McElroy, S. L., and Nixon, R. A. Possible synergism between fluoxetine and lithium in refractory depression. *Am. J. Psychiatry* 145 : 1292, 1988.

Price, L. H., Charney, D. S., and Heninger, G. R. Variability of response to lithium augmentation in refractory depression. *Am. J. Psychiatry* 143 : 1387, 1986.

Alcoholism

de la Fuente, J. R., Morse, R. M., Niven, R. G., and Ilstrup, D. M. A controlled study of lithium carbonate in the treatment of alcoholism. *Mayo Clin. Proc.* 64 : 177, 1989.

Dorus, W., Ostrow, D. G., Anton, R., et al. Lithium treatment of depressed and nondepressed alcoholics. *J.A.M.A.* 262 : 1646, 1989.

Fawcett, J., Clark, D. C., Aagesen, C. A., et al. A double-blind, placebo-controlled trial of lithium carbonate therapy for alcoholism. *Arch. Gen. Psychiatry* 44 : 248, 1987.

Other Indications for Lithium

Schiff, H. B., Sabin, T. D., Geller, A., et al. Lithium in aggressive behavior. *Am. J. Psychiatry* 139 : 1346, 1982.

Other Issues in Management of Bipolar Patients

Kane, J. M. The role of neuroleptics in manic-depressive illness. *J. Clin. Psychiatry* 49(Suppl.) : 12, 1988.

Post, R. M., Roy-Byrne, P. P., and Uhde, T. W. Graphic representation of the life course of illness in patients with affective disorder. *Am. J. Psychiatry* 145 : 844, 1988.

Shukla, S., Mukherjee, S., and Decina, P. Lithium in the treatment of bipolar disorders associated with epilepsy: An open study. *J. Clin. Psychopharmacol.* 8 : 201, 1988.

Wehr, T. A., and Goodwin, F. K. Rapid cycling in manic-depressives induced by tricyclic antidepressants. *Arch. Gen. Psychiatry* 37 : 555, 1979.

Wehr, T. A., and Goodwin, F. K. Can antidepressants cause mania and worsen the course of affective illness? *Am. J. Psychiatry* 144 : 1403, 1987.

Wehr, T. A., Sack, D. A., Rosenthal, N. E., and Cowdry, R. W. Rapid cycling affective disorder: Contributing factors and treatment responses in 51 patients. *Am. J. Psychiatry* 145 : 179, 1988.

Method of Use

Cooper, T. B., and Simpson, G. M. The 24-hour lithium level as a prognosticator of dosage requirements: A two-year follow-up study. *Am. J. Psychiatry* 133 : 440, 1976.

Jefferson, J. W., Greist, J. H., Clagnaz, P. J., et al. Effect of strenuous exercise on serum lithium level in man. *Am. J. Psychiatry* 139 : 1593, 1982.

Perry, P. J., Dunner, F. J., Hahn, R. L., et al. Lithium kinetics in single daily dosing. *Acta Psychiatr. Scand.* 64 : 281, 1981.

Post, R. M., Roy-Byrne, P. P., and Uhde, T. W. Graphic representation of the life course of illness in patients with affective disorder. *Am. J. Psychiatry* 145 : 844, 1988.

Side Effects and Toxicity

Acute Lithium Intoxication

Schou, M. The Recognition and Management of Lithium Intoxication. In F. N. Johnson (ed.), *Handbook of Lithium Therapy*. Lancaster, England: MTP Press, 1980.

Simard, M., Gumbiner, B., Lee, A., et al. Lithium carbonate intoxication: A case report and review of the literature. *Arch. Intern. Med.* 149 : 36, 1989.

Lithium and the Kidney

Battle, D. C., von Riotte, A. B., Gavira, M., and Grupp, M. Amelioration of polyuria by amiloride in patients receiving long-term lithium therapy. *N. Engl. J. Med.* 312 : 408, 1985.

Bowen, R. C., Grof, P., and Grof, E. Less frequent lithium administration and lower urine volume. *Am. J. Psychiatry* 148 : 189, 1991.

De Paulo, J. R., Jr., Correa, E. I., and Sapir, D. G. Renal function and lithium: A longitudinal study. *Am. J. Psychiatry* 143 : 892, 1986.

Hetmar, O., Brun, C., Clemmsen, L., et al. Lithium: Long-term effects on the kidney: II. Structural changes. *J. Psychiatr. Res.* 21 : 279, 1987.

Hetmar, O., Clemmsen, L., Ladefoged, J., and Rafaelsen, O. J. Lithium: Long-term effects on the kidney: III. Prospective study. *Acta Psychiatr. Scand.* 75 : 251, 1987.

Kosten, T. R., and Forrest, J. N. Treatment of severe lithium-induced polyuria with amiloride. *Am. J. Psychiatry* 143 : 1563, 1986.

Plenge, P., and Raaelson, O. J. Lithium treatment: Does the kidney prefer one daily dose instead of two? *Acta Psychiatr. Scand.* 66 : 121, 1982.

Wood, I. K., Parmelee, D. X., Foreman, J. W. Lithium-induced nephrotic syndrome. *Am. J. Psychiatry* 146 : 84, 1989.

Neurologic Toxicities

Apte, S. N., and Langston, J. W. Permanent neurological deficits due to lithium toxicity. *Ann. Neurol.* 13 : 452, 1983.

Engelsmann, F., Katz, J., Ghadirian, A. M., and Schacter, D. Lithium and memory: A long-term follow-up study. *J. Clin. Psychopharmacol.* 8 : 207, 1988.

Joffe, R. T., MacDonald, C., and Kutcher, S. P. Lack of differential cognitive effects of lithium and carbamazepine in bipolar affective disorder. *J. Clin. Psychopharmacol.* 8 : 425, 1988.

Saul, R. F., Hamberger, H. A., and Selhorst, J. B. Pseudotumor cerebri secondary to lithium carbonate. *J.A.M.A.* 253 : 2869, 1985.

Schou, M. Long-lasting neurological sequelae after lithium intoxication. *Acta Psychiatr. Scand.* 70 : 594, 1984.

Other Toxicities

Deandrea, D., Walker, N., Mehlmauer, M., and White, K. Dermatological reactions to lithium: A critical review of the literature. *J. Clin. Psychopharmacol.* 2 : 199, 1982.

Franks, R. D., Dubovsky, S. L., Lifshitz, M., et al. Long-term lithium carbonate therapy causes hyperparathyroidism. *Arch. Gen. Psychiatry* 39 : 1074, 1982.

Garland, E. J., Remick, R. A., and Zis, A. P. Weight gain with antidepressants and lithium. *J. Clin. Psychopharmacol.* 8 : 323, 1988.

Lyman, G. H., Williams, C. C., Dinwoodie, W. R., and Schocken, D. D. Sudden death in cancer patients receiving lithium. *J. Clin. Oncol.* 2 : 1270, 1984.

Mitchell, J. E., and Mackenzie, T. B. Cardiac effects of lithium therapy in man: A review. *J. Clin. Psychiatry* 43 : 47, 1982.

Susman, V. L., and Adonizio, G. Reintroduction of neuroleptic malignant syndrome by lithium. *J. Clin. Psychopharmacol.* 7 : 339, 1987.

Yassa, R., Saunders, A., Nastase, C., and Camile, Y. Lithium-induced thyroid disorders: A prevalence study. *J. Clin. Psychiatry* 48 : 14, 1988.

Drug Interactions

Miller, F., and Meninger, J. Lithium-neuroleptic neurotoxicity is dose dependent. *J. Clin. Psychopharmacol.* 7 : 89, 1987.

Ragheb, M. The clinical significance of lithium-nonsteroidal anti-inflammatory drug interactions. *J. Clin. Psychopharmacol.* 10 : 350, 1990.

Use in Pregnancy

Cohen, L. S., Friedman, J. M., Jefferson, J. W., et al. A reevaluation of risk of in utero exposure to lithium. *J. A. M. A.* 271 : 146, 1994.

Zalstein, E., Koren, G., Einarson, T., and Freedom, R. M. A case control study on the association between 1st trimester exposure to lithium and Ebstein's anomaly. *Am. J. Cardiol.* 65 : 817, 1990.

5

Psychiatric Uses of Anticonvulsants

This chapter focuses on the psychiatric uses of anticonvulsants. Epilepsy and other neurologic disorders are mentioned only briefly because a full discussion would occupy an entire volume. Two anticonvulsants have proved particularly useful in the treatment of bipolar disorder (Fig. 5-1), and other psychiatric uses of anticonvulsants have been contemplated. Carbamazepine was the first anticonvulsant used to treat mania, but many clinicians now believe that valproic acid is more promising. Valproic acid is becoming a widely accepted agent in the treatment of bipolar disorder. Carbamazepine is also a useful treatment for bipolar disorder and has been tried in several other conditions. Both valproic acid and carbamazepine have a similar profile of effectiveness in bipolar disorder to lithium in that they demonstrate greater efficacy in treating and preventing manias than depressions.

Phenytoin and the barbiturates do not appear to possess mood-stabilizing properties that would make them useful in the treatment of bipolar disorder. Several recently approved anticonvulsants have not been adequately studied for psychiatric applications. Clonazepam, a benzodiazepine with high enough potency and a long enough half-life to be used as an anticonvulsant, is effective in panic disorder and is a useful adjunct in the treatment of some patients with bipolar disorder or other psychotic conditions who require greater anxiolysis or sedation than is provided by their primary therapeutic agents. Clonazepam is fully discussed in Chapter 6.

Lithium remains the first-choice treatment for bipolar disorder; nonetheless, approximately 30% of bipolar patients either have a poor response to lithium or cannot tolerate it. Given the side effects of antipsychotic drugs and the long-term risk of tardive dyskinesia with standard antipsychotics (which may be elevated in patients with mood disorders), the use of antipsychotics in bipolar disorder should be minimized if possible. Clozapine is not likely to cause tardive dyskinesia but has many side effects that adversely affect quality of life. Electroconvulsive therapy (ECT) is effective in the treatment of acute mania and depression; however, it does not appear to be a viable long-term treatment. Thus, the development of anticonvulsants as alternatives to lithium is quite welcome.

VALPROIC ACID

Valproic acid is effective in the control of absence (petit mal), myoclonic, and generalized tonic-clonic seizures. It is less effective in partial seizures with or without complex symptomatology. An increasing number of well-designed studies suggest that it is effective for bipolar disorder both as a single agent and in combination with lithium.

Pharmacology

Valproic acid is available in several different preparations and dosage forms (Table 5-1). Whatever form is chosen, valproic acid is the active compound in serum. Valproic acid is available in capsule or syrup form. Divalproex sodium is an enteric-coated form that contains equal parts valproic acid and sodium valproate. Valproic acid is rapidly absorbed after oral administration, achieving peak

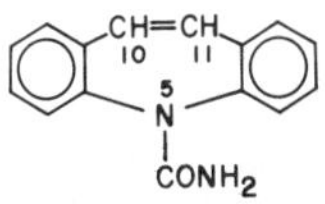

Fig. 5-1. Anticonvulsants. Chemical structures of carbamazepine and valproic acid.

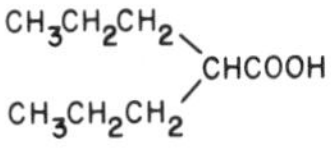

Table 5-1. Available preparations of valproic acid and carbamazepine

Form	Brand Name	How Supplied
Valproic acid	Depakene	250-mg capsules
	Depakene	250-mg/5-ml syrup
	Valproic Acid	250-mg capsules
Divalproex sodium	Depakote	125-, 250-, 500-mg tablets
	Depakote	125-mg sprinkle capsules
Carbamazepine	Atretol	200-mg tablet
	Tegretol	100-, 200-mg tablets
	Tegretol	100-mg/5-ml suspension
	Carbamazepine	200-mg tablets
	Carbamazepine	100-mg chewable tablets

levels in 1–2 hours if taken on an empty stomach and in 4–5 hours if taken with food. Divalproex sodium is more slowly absorbed, reaching peak serum concentrations in 3–8 hours.

In plasma, valproic acid is 80–95% protein-bound. It is rapidly metabolized by the liver; it has no known active metabolites. Interactions with other protein-bound or hepatically metabolized drugs occur. Valproic acid has a short elimination half-life of approximately 8 hours, thus 3 times daily dosing is usually recommended for epilepsy; the need for divided dosing in bipolar disorder has not been established.

There is a poor correlation between serum levels and antimanic effects, but levels in the range of 50–150 μg/ml are generally required. Blood levels are measured by immunoassay or gas chromatography.

The **mechanism of action** in both bipolar disorder and epilepsy is unknown, but valproic acid is known to increase levels of gamma-aminobutyric acid (GABA), the principal inhibitory neurotransmitter in the brain. Experimentally, it blocks the convulsive effects of the $GABA_A$ receptor antagonists, picrotoxin and bicuculline.

Psychiatric Indications

Bipolar Disorder

The best established psychiatric use of valproic acid is in the treatment of acute mania. Only a small number of well-designed studies have examined the efficacy of valproic acid for acute mania; only one of these compared valproic acid to lithium. Based on these, on earlier nonblind studies, and on clinical experience, valproic acid appears to be effective for acute mania and may be as effective as lithium. Based on small studies and case reports, some lithium-refractory patients respond to valproic acid alone or in combination with lithium, carbamazepine, typical antipsychotic drugs, or clozapine.

There are no double-blind placebo-controlled studies of valproic acid for acute bipolar depression or for bipolar prophylaxis. Based on open studies, it appears that when used for prophylaxis, valproic acid is more effective in preventing manic than depressive recurrences. Open studies and anecdotal clinical data do not currently support the use of valproic acid as an antidepressant. However, valproic acid may have a role in preventing mania in bipolar patients being treated concomitantly with an antidepressant.

In general clinical use, the experience with valproic acid has been inconsistent, but that likely reflects the treatment-refractory nature of many of the patients who receive it. There are credible reports of valproic acid succeeding for patients who did not respond to either lithium or carbamazepine.

Schizoaffective Disorder

There are no well-designed trials to study the use of valproic acid in schizoaffective patients, but open trials and case reports suggest that an empirical trial of valproic acid may be reasonable for patients who have recurrent manic-like episodes not adequately treated with lithium. There are no data to support trials of valproic acid in well-diagnosed schizophrenic patients or schizoaffective patients whose episodes of mood disorder are exclusively depressive. Use of mood stabilizers in schizoaffective and schizophreniform disorders are more fully discussed in Chapter 4.

Therapeutic Use

There is no standardized workup prior to initiation of valproic acid therapy, but it is optimal to obtain a general medical history and examination, with particular attention to other drugs used by the patient and any history of liver disease or bleeding disorder. Ideally, baseline liver function tests (LFTs) and a complete blood count (CBC) with platelets will also be obtained. Valproic acid should not be administered to patients with known liver disease.

Valproic acid therapy should be initiated slowly to minimize side effects. A first test dose of 250 mg is best given with a meal. Gradually the dosage can be increased to 250 mg tid over several days as gastrointestinal symptoms and sedation allow. Further dosage increases, probably up to 1800 mg/day, can be made as needed to control symptoms. Optimal blood levels for both seizure disorders and mania are debated but appear to be in the range of 50–150 µg/ml. Blood levels may be obtained weekly until the patient is stable. Many clinicians also obtain LFTs and a CBC at the same time. Antimanic effects are generally seen within 1–2 weeks of achieving target levels.

In stable, asymptomatic patients, blood levels, LFTs, and a CBC may be obtained every 6 months. However, new onset of side effects after stable therapy has been achieved should prompt immediate measurement of drug levels and additional appropriate workup. For example, late onset of nausea, anorexia, or fatigue is an indication for obtaining levels and LFTs, including ammonia levels.

Use in Pregnancy

Valproic acid has not been as well studied in pregnancy as several other anticonvulsants, but it has been associated with major congenital malformations including spina bifida. Alterations in clotting function may also pose risks to mother and fetus later in pregnancy and at parturition. Alternative treatments for mania that appear to be safer include ECT and high-potency antipsychotic drugs. (See also Chap. 4 for concerns about lithium in pregnancy.) Valproic acid is secreted in breast milk at concentrations 1–10% of serum concentration. The effect on the developing child is unknown.

Side Effects and Toxicity

Minor side effects are common at the start of treatment with valproic acid and are often transient. These include gastrointestinal effects (including nausea, vomiting, anorexia, heartburn, and diarrhea), sedation, tremor, and ataxia (Table 5-2). Administration with food or use of enteric-coated preparations, such as divalproex, may help diminish gastrointestinal effects. Histamine H_2 receptor blockers such as ranitidine may also decrease upper gastrointestinal distress but risk possible drug interactions. Approximately one-half of those treated initially experience some degree of sedation. This tends to diminish with chronic use. Sedation may become a severe problem when valproic acid is coadministered with other anticonvulsants, especially phenobarbital (which is not used for bipolar disorder). Valproic acid appears to cause mild impairment of cognitive function with chronic use; in this regard it is slightly worse than carbamazepine, but superior to phenytoin or barbiturates.

The other common side effects of valproic acid are alopecia and weight gain.

Table 5-2. Side effects and toxicity of valproic acid

Common side effects
    Gastrointestinal: nausea, vomiting, anorexia, heartburn, diarrhea
    Hematologic: thrombocytopenia, platelet dysfunction
    Hepatic: benign elevation of transaminases
    Neurologic: sedation, tremor, ataxia
    Other: alopecia, weight gain
Less common side effects
    Hematologic: bleeding tendency
    Metabolic: hyperammonemia
    Neurologic: incoordination, asterixis, stupor, coma, behavioral
        automatisms
Serious idiosyncratic side effects
    Hepatitis/hepatic failure
    Pancreatitis
    Drug rashes, including erythema multiforme

Hepatotoxicity

Valproic acid may cause transient dose-dependent asymptomatic rises in aspartate and alanine transaminases in 15–30% of patients, which are an indication for monitoring but not for stopping treatment. These laboratory abnormalities are generally maximal during the first 3 months of treatment. Isolated hyperammonemia, which may be accompanied by confusion or lethargy, has been reported rarely. These hepatic effects usually improve with decreased dosage. Rare cases of fatal hepatotoxicity associated with valproate have been reported. Between 1978 and 1984, 37 cases were discovered. All but one patient had medical conditions in addition to the seizure disorder for which valproate was being prescribed, such as mental retardation, developmental delay, congenital abnormalities, or other neurologic disorders. Between 1985 and 1986, the rate of fatal hepatotoxicity was 2.5 in 100,000 patients. For patients receiving valproate as their only anticonvulsant drug, the rate of fatal hepatotoxicity was 0.85 in 100,000 patients. No hepatic fatalities have been reported in patients above age 10 receiving valproate as their only anticonvulsant. There is inadequate experience with valproate-lithium combinations or in populations with psychiatric rather than seizure disorders to comment on the relative risk of hepatic toxicity in psychiatric use, but the risk appears to be very low, and certainly far lower than the risk to life from undertreated bipolar disorder. Minor elevations in hepatic transaminases are not a warning sign. Should significant liver function abnormalities or symptoms of hepatitis occur (e.g., malaise, anorexia, jaundice, abdominal pain, or edema), the drug should be immediately discontinued and the patient carefully monitored.

Neurotoxicity

As noted previously, sedation is the most serious problem, and hand tremor is the most common long-term neurologic side effect. If troublesome, these side effects generally diminish if the dosage is decreased. There are anecdotal reports of tremor responding to beta-adrenergic blockers, such as propranolol (as in the case of lithium tremor; see Chap. 7), but beta-blockers have been associated with their own central nervous system side effects, including depression-like symptoms. Ataxia may occur at higher doses of valproic acid. Rarely, asterixis, stupor, coma, and behavioral automatisms have been reported.

Hematologic Toxicity

Valproic acid can cause thrombocytopenia or platelet dysfunction, but only rarely is it associated with bleeding complications. This effect is usually only observed in patients on high doses. Patients on valproate should have their platelet count and bleeding time checked before any surgery.

Other Serious Idiosyncratic Toxicities

Rarely, hemorrhagic pancreatitis may occur, usually in the first 6 months of treatment, and may be fatal. Agranulocytosis is also a rare idiosyncratic side effect. Drug rashes, including erythema multiforme, have also been reported.

Serious Dose-Related Toxicities and Overdoses

Excessive serum levels may occur in the context of drug-drug interactions or intentional overdose. The symptoms of overdose include severe neurologic symptoms. Overdose with valproic acid can be treated with hemodialysis. Only very rare fatalities have been reported.

Drug Interactions

Valproic acid may have pharmacodynamic interactions with other psychotropic drugs, including carbamazepine, lithium, and antipsychotic drugs, producing combined central nervous system toxicity. Whenever multiple psychotropic drugs are coadministered, patients must be monitored for deterioration of mental status.

Valproic acid also produces pharmacokinetic interactions with many drugs. It inhibits the metabolism of drugs that are oxidized by the liver; thus it may increase levels of cyclic antidepressants and possibly selective serotonin reuptake inhibitors (SSRIs), phenytoin, phenobarbital, and other drugs. Valproic acid may also increase the effective levels of other protein-bound drugs, or conversely, it may be displaced from protein binding by drugs such as aspirin, precipitating valproic acid toxicity. Thus patients who must take other protein-bound drugs, such as warfarin, must be monitored closely at the initiation of combined therapy.

Valproic acid concentrations may be decreased by drugs, such as carbamazepine, that induce hepatic microsomal enzymes. Its concentrations may be increased by drugs, such as SSRIs, that inhibit hepatic microsomal enzymes.

It should also be noted that valproic acid is partially eliminated in the urine as a ketometabolite, which may lead to false interpretations of urine ketone tests.

CARBAMAZEPINE

Carbamazepine is an iminostilbene anticonvulsant that is structurally similar to the tricyclic antidepressant imipramine. It is generally considered to be the drug of first choice in the treatment of partial epilepsy with or without complex symptomatology; it is also effective for primary generalized seizures. Carbamazepine is also the treatment of choice in trigeminal neuralgia and is used in other neuropathic pain syndromes that have a lancinating component.

Several reports in the neurologic literature suggested that carbamazepine improved mood symptoms in patients treated for epilepsy. It was first reported as a primary treatment for manic depressive illness in Japan in the early 1970s. Since that time, many studies of carbamazepine for acute mania have been performed, although few have been well designed. Carbamazepine is more effective than placebo for acute mania. It remains uncertain whether it is as effective as lithium. It appears to be useful for some patients in long-term bipolar prophylaxis, but its general utility for this indication has not been established, and some reports have suggested diminishing effectiveness over time. On the basis of small studies and case reports, some investigators have suggested that carbamazepine may be particularly effective for patients with forms of bipolar disorder that are often relatively refractory to lithium (i.e., patients with mixed bipolar symptoms [both manic and depressed symptoms present], dysphoric mania, and rapid-cycling bipolar disorder). Carbamazepine is now under study for a variety of psychiatric disorders other than bipolar disorder.

Pharmacology

Carbamazepine is available for oral administration as 100-mg and 200-mg tablets and as a suspension (see Table 5-1). No parenteral forms are available. Its absorption is slow and erratic, with peak levels usually achieved in 4–8 hours, but occasionally later. Slow-release forms appear to produce more stable serum concentrations than regular tablets. Carbamazepine is poorly soluble in gastrointestinal fluids; after oral administration, 15–25% is excreted unchanged in the feces. The effect of food on absorption does not appear to be clinically significant. In the blood it is 65–80% protein-bound.

Blood levels can be measured by gas-liquid chromatography, high-pressure liquid chromatography, and immunoassays. Therapeutic levels for epilepsy are in the range of 4–12 μg/ml (core range 6–10 μg/ml), with the lower end of the range typically effective for tonic-clonic seizures and the higher end effective for partial seizures with or without tonic-clonic seizures. For bipolar disorder, initial studies suggested that blood levels in the range of 8–12 μg/ml corresponded with therapeutic efficacy. More recently this correlation has appeared less certain. A therapeutic effect is unlikely with a level of less than 4 μg/ml; however, many clinicians no longer recommend use of blood levels to titrate efficacy in bipolar disorder.

Carbamazepine is metabolized by the liver. Its 10-, 11-epoxide metabolite (which may reach levels 20% as high as the parent compound) is an effective anticonvulsant; it is unknown whether it is also an active antimanic agent. The elimination half-life of carbamazepine in a single dose in healthy volunteers is 18–55 hours; however, with repeat dosing the half-life decreases to 5–20 hours (longer in the elderly). This reduction in half-life with repeat dosing is due to the drug inducing its own metabolism by hepatic P450 enzymes. This induction may be clinically significant. An oral dose, which is effective early in therapy, may become ineffective due to falling levels after several weeks. This autoinduction effect generally plateaus within 3–5 weeks. Carbamazepine metabolism also can be induced by other drugs, especially the anticonvulsants, phenytoin, phenobarbital, and primidone, resulting in lower serum levels.

Mechanism of Action

Carbamazepine has two known mechanisms that may be relevant to its antiepileptic effect. Opening of voltage-sensitive sodium channels is central to the mechanism of neuronal action potentials. These channels become temporarily inactive after use. Carbamazepine binds to an inactivated state of sodium channels, resulting in use-dependent and voltage-dependent block. Thus, carbamazepine inhibits repetitive firing of action potentials. This effect of carbamazepine seems particularly to affect sodium channels localized on neuronal cell bodies. Carbamazepine also appears to block presynaptic sodium channels, thus inhibiting depolarization of presynaptic terminals in response to action potentials propagated down the axon. Since the depolarizing effect of the sodium action potential is blocked, voltage-gated calcium channels are secondarily inhibited. The result is decreased calcium entry into the presynaptic terminal and a decrement in neurotransmitter release. Mechanisms of this type could have widespread effects on neural function in addition to treating epilepsy. Their relevance to mood disorder is not known.

There are a variety of animal models in epilepsy. Carbamazepine appears to be the most active anticonvulsant in blocking the development of seizures in the kindling model. Kindling involves the repetitive application of subthreshold electrical or chemical stimuli to produce an autonomous epileptic focus. The effectiveness of carbamazepine in this model has led to a great deal of theorizing that mood disorders and other psychiatric disorders may represent a kindling process. Although no convincing mechanistic models of kindling in mood disorders have emerged to date, speculation about kindling has produced valuable reexaminations concerning the course of psychiatric disorders, focusing attention on the observation that episodes may become more frequent and more autonomous (less related to environmental precipitants) over time in a subset of patients.

Indications

Acute Mania

In both published studies and clinical practice, carbamazepine appears to be effective in the treatment of acute mania; however, the number of patients studied in placebo-controlled double-blind fashion remains small, and many study populations are atypical. Thus carbamazepine appears to be effective for acute mania, but it is not clear whether it is as effective as lithium or even valproate.

At present, the effective oral dose for each patient must be determined empirically by upward dosage titration, using the attainment of therapeutic effects and the emergence of side effects to guide dosing. For acute mania, an average effective dose is approximately 1000 mg/day (range 200–1800 mg/day). After a therapeutic dosage is established, patients must be carefully observed because after several weeks carbamazepine may induce its own metabolism, requiring a dosage increase. Therapeutic dosage levels for bipolar disorder have not been established; many clinicians use the levels that have been established for epilepsy as a general guide.

If an episode of mania is mild, carbamazepine alone may be adequate treatment. For severe manic episodes, however, carbamazepine is usually begun along with an antipsychotic drug and/or a benzodiazepine to gain more rapid control of manic behavior. Neuroleptic doses equivalent to haloperidol, 8–10 mg/day, are usually effective. Higher doses carry a risk of worsened side effects without strong evidence of added benefit. If possible, the antipsychotic medication should be tapered and discontinued after the acute symptoms have resolved, and the patient should be maintained on carbamazepine alone. Some patients who do not respond to lithium or carbamazepine as single agents respond to the combination at full therapeutic doses. The most compelling evidence for this synergy comes from longitudinal "on-off-on" trials, but only small numbers of patients have been studied, generally in an unblinded fashion. Similarly, combined therapy with carbamazepine and valproic acid has been reported effective in some refractory patients with acute mania.

Bipolar Prophylaxis

Several studies have suggested that carbamazepine may be effective for prophylaxis against recurrences in bipolar disorder, but there is a paucity of placebo-controlled or double-blind studies. Taken together, the published studies and clinical experience underscore the point that long-term prophylactic use of carbamazepine in bipolar disorder is less well established than its use in acute mania. For example, while one unblinded prospective study of lithium-refractory patients found carbamazepine to be effective in bipolar prophylaxis as a single agent in some patients and in combination with lithium in others over a mean of 20.2 months (Stuppaeck et al., 1990), a retrospective study found carbamazepine to be relatively ineffective after 3–4 years in lithium-refractory patients (Frankenburg et al., 1988). Interpretation of these contrasting studies is made difficult by serious methodologic problems in each report. Clearly more research is necessary, but for the present, it is reasonable to use carbamazepine for long-term prophylaxis either singly or with lithium in patients who have been treated with that regimen for their acute mania. The effectiveness of carbamazepine or any other prophylactic agent can only be judged after a sufficiently long period of time to compare the patient's rate of cycling on carbamazepine with the patient's prior rate of cycling. This will vary depending on the patient's base rate. Dosage for prophylaxis is not established; it is reasonable to use the same dosage that is effective for the patient during acute manic episodes and to decrease the dosage only if side effects may limit therapy. The current evidence suggests that carbamazepine may be more effective in prophylaxis against manic than against depressive recurrences.

Rapid-Cycling Bipolar Disorder

Lithium is less effective for rapidly cycling patients (i.e., those with more than three cycles per year) than for patients with more typical bipolar disorder (see Chap. 4). Despite the lack of clear proof that carbamazepine is effective for long-term bipolar prophylaxis, there is some evidence that it may be more effective than lithium for rapid cyclers. In a small, partly blinded longitudinal trial, Post and associates (1983) compared the course of illness of seven rapidly cycling, lithium-resistant bipolar patients before and after administration of carbamazepine. The patients were followed for an average of 1.7 years on carbamazepine, with a decrease in total (manic and depressive) recurrences from 16.4 to 5.6 per year. It is important to note that although carbamazepine improved the course of rapid-cycling illness, it did not suppress all affective recurrences. It may take 6 months to a year to judge the efficacy of carbamazepine for this population.

Acute Depression

Both controlled studies and clinical practice suggest that carbamazepine is effective only for a small minority of patients with acute depression, whether unipolar or bipolar. The rate of improvement with carbamazepine is no better than the placebo rate in older antidepressant trials; however, some patients appear to have a true response based on "on-off-on" trial designs, with placebo substituted in blinded fashion after initial carbamazepine-associated improvement. Enough patients have worsened on placebo and improved again on carbamazepine to suggest that even though the number of responders is not great, some of those who improve are true rather than placebo responders. An average antidepressant dosage is approximately 1000 mg/day of carbamazepine. Carbamazepine has also been associated with the onset of depression. In a study of carbamazepine for the treatment of borderline personality disorder, 3 of 17 patients developed melancholia that remitted with discontinuation of carbamazepine.

In clinical practice, carbamazepine should not be considered in the normal treatment algorithm for depression. If used in depression, carbamazepine should be given in at least a 2- to 4-week trial because the evidence suggests that it works more slowly in depression than in mania.

Psychiatric Symptoms Secondary to Seizure Disorders

SECONDARY AFFECTIVE SYMPTOMS. Many patients with complex partial seizures have secondary affective instability and depression. Carbamazepine, which is the drug of choice for this form of epilepsy, appears to produce improvement in related affective symptomatology. The effect often parallels optimal seizure control.

Some epileptic patients remain depressed despite good seizure control. In treating these patients, it should be recalled that cyclic antidepressants and bupropion lower the seizure threshold (maprotiline, clomipramine, and bupropion appear to have the greatest likelihood of inducing seizures and are best avoided); however, SSRIs do not. In addition, carbamazepine and other anticonvulsants may induce the metabolism of antidepressants, and SSRIs may inhibit the metabolism of anticonvulsants. If depression is severe enough to require treatment, an SSRI or possibly venlafaxine should be added. When antidepressants are used, the patient's neurologic status and serum anticonvulsant levels should be closely monitored.

SECONDARY PSYCHOTIC SYMPTOMS. Psychotic symptoms can be produced by complex partial seizures in two ways: as an ictal symptom or chronically as a late sequela to this form of epilepsy. Anticonvulsants, including carbamazepine, are far more effective in treating psychotic symptoms due to a seizure (by suppressing seizure activity) than in treating the chronic psychotic syndrome of long-term complex partial epilepsy. The cause of this latter syndrome is unknown.

Treatment of secondary psychotic symptoms that do not respond to anticonvulsants is best attempted by adding an antipsychotic drug to the regimen. High-potency antipsychotic agents, such as haloperidol, appear to have little effect on the seizure threshold. Low-potency antipsychotics, such as chlorpromazine or thioridazine, may lower the seizure threshold and should be avoided. Carbamazepine induces hepatic metabolic enzymes and may therefore lower the blood levels of antipsychotics. Thus higher antipsychotic doses (perhaps as high as 20 mg of haloperidol) may occasionally be necessary, although in most patients dosages of 10 mg/day are likely to be effective.

Whether carbamazepine treatment early in the course of complex partial epilepsy can prevent late psychotic sequelae is currently a matter of speculation. A small minority of seizure patients with secondary psychotic symptoms develop a worsening pattern of psychosis when their seizures are markedly decreased in frequency or eliminated. If these symptoms are severe and prove resistant to antipsychotic treatment, optimal therapy may require that the patient be allowed to have infrequent seizures. It must be stressed that such patients are rare and are probably best cared for by physicians with experience in the treatment of complex partial seizure disorders.

Schizophrenia

There have been reports that carbamazepine confers additive benefits when used with antipsychotic drugs in the treatment of acutely agitated schizophrenic patients. These studies suggest that carbamazepine may be helpful in calming agitation and decreasing aggressive behavior, but further confirmatory data are needed. In clinical practice, carbamazepine might be added to an antipsychotic drug as an innovative trial in acutely agitated schizophrenics otherwise refractory to treatment. Before doing so, however, it is important to be sure that the agitation is not due to neuroleptic-induced akathisia. A short trial of benzodiazepines (e.g., lorazepam, 1–2 mg tid prn) is a more conservative approach than the use of carbamazepine and should be attempted first.

There is little evidence to suggest that carbamazepine is useful in long-term maintenance treatment of well-diagnosed schizophrenics. A recent case report describes a striking exacerbation of psychotic symptoms in two chronic schizophrenic patients following abrupt termination of a carbamazepine trial after the trial was deemed a failure; thus it would be prudent to taper carbamazepine if used in this population even if it had no apparent effect.

Atypical Psychoses: Schizoaffective and Schizophreniform Disorders

Use of mood stabilizers in schizoaffective and schizophreniform disorders are more fully discussed in Chapter 4. Based on clinical reports, mood stabilizers, including lithium, valproate, and carbamazepine, may be indicated for schizoaffective patients, especially those with manic symptoms, or for schizophreniform patients. On this basis, a trial of carbamazepine might be indicated in selected schizoaffective or schizophreniform patients who are unresponsive to or intolerant of lithium.

Episodic Dyscontrol Syndromes

There are both anecdotal reports and small studies of carbamazepine use in treating impulsive and aggressive behavior in nonpsychotic patients. For example, in one double-blind crossover trial in borderline patients with prominent histories of dyscontrol, carbamazepine decreased dyscontrol in 10 of 11 patients and was more effective than alprazolam, trifluoperazine, or tranylcypromine for this indication (Gardner and Cowdry, 1986). Other medications proposed for dyscontrol are lithium, valproate, and propranolol. Propranolol has been found effective in some open studies, especially in patients with brain damage or dementia (see Chap. 7). Antipsychotic drugs are often tried for dyscontrol but are generally ineffective unless the patient is psychotic, and they also pose the risk of tardive dyskinesia. At present, no pharmacologic agent has been shown to be effective for the longitudinal treatment of dyscontrol. Each treatment represents an empirical trial. The risk of toxicity from carbamazepine or any other drug must be judged against the frequency and severity of dyscontrol on an individual basis.

Neuropathic Pain

Pain may develop in response to an injury to peripheral or central sensory afferents. Because of damage to the nociceptive pathways, there is generally some loss of normal pain sensation (hypalgesia), but severe neuropathic pain may follow after a delay. Such pain may be produced by processes such as amputation, nerve avulsion, cordotomy, or peripheral neuropathy. Phantom limb pain, causalgia, postherpetic neuralgia, and thalamic pain are all forms of neuropathic pain.

The symptoms of neuropathic pain may include persistent burning or unprovoked paroxysms of lancinating pain referred to the deafferented region. Patients may also describe dysesthesias (e.g., pins and needles, numbness or tingling, or formication, a feeling of insects crawling on the skin). In addition, mildly noxious stimuli may provoke severe pain in the region (hyperpathia), and even innocuous stimuli applied to this region may produce perverted sensations or severe pain (allodynia).

Carbamazepine is the drug of choice in the treatment of trigeminal neuralgia (tic douloureux) and a related syndrome that occurs in the distribution of the glossopharyngeal nerve. It appears to be somewhat more effective in these conditions than phenytoin, although the latter is also effective. The high-potency benzodiazepine clonazepam may also have some role in these conditions. Carbamazepine may also be effective for neuropathic pain due to diabetic neuropathy, multiple sclerosis, postherpetic neuralgia, and other conditions, especially if there is a paroxysmal, lancinating component. In these latter conditions, however, most clinicians begin with a tricyclic antidepressant (see Chap. 3). Carbamazepine is begun at low doses (e.g., 100 mg bid) and slowly increased until relief occurs (usually in the range of 400–800 mg/day).

As Detoxification Agent

Several open and controlled trials have suggested that carbamazepine is effective for alcohol withdrawal. One randomized double-blind study of 86 men with severe alcohol withdrawal found carbamazepine, 800 mg/day, as effective as oxazepam, 120 mg/day, with no difference in side effects (Malcolm et al., 1989). Given the long track record of safety and efficacy for benzodiazepines, more study would be required before carbamazepine could be recommended as a detoxification agent for ethanol.

A small number of reports have also suggested that carbamazepine, 200–800 mg/day, may be a useful adjunct for withdrawal from alprazolam and other benzodiazepines. While this strategy may aid individual patients, a large controlled study failed to show evidence of efficacy. Should this approach be attempted, there are little data to guide the clinician on the appropriate duration of carbamazepine treatment to maintain patients benzodiazepine-free. In one trial, patients were placed on carbamazepine, 400 mg, for 1–2 weeks prior to detoxification at a rate of 25% per week. Carbamazepine was maintained for 14 days after the benzodiazepine taper ended (Schweizer et al., 1991).

Seizures

The use of carbamazepine as an anticonvulsant (Table 5-3) is fully reviewed in other sources. The method of administration and side

Table 5-3.   Use of carbamazepine for seizure disorders

Effective	*Ineffective*
Simple partial	Generalized absence
Complex partial	
Generalized tonic-clonic	
Mixed seizure patterns that include complex partial, tonic-clonic, or other partial or generalized seizures	

effect monitoring is the same for epilepsy as is described below for psychiatric disorders.

Therapeutic Use

Preliminary Workup

Patients who are candidates for carbamazepine treatment should have a medical history and physical examination with emphasis on prior history of blood dyscrasias or liver disease. Laboratory tests should include a CBC with platelets and liver and renal function tests. Patients with hematologic abnormalities should be considered at high risk for serious blood dyscrasias if treated with carbamazepine; they therefore deserve closer follow-up than usual. Patients with significant hepatic disease should not receive this drug unless there are no better alternatives; they should be started on one-third to one-half the normal starting dosage with longer than usual time (5–7 days) between dosage adjustments.

Beginning Carbamazepine

In patients over the age of 12, carbamazepine is begun at 200 mg bid. The dosage is increased by no more than 200 mg/day until therapeutic levels are achieved. The clinical situation determines how aggressively the dosage may be increased. In hospitalized patients with acute mania, the dosage might be increased daily in 200-mg increments up to 800–1000 mg unless side effects develop, with slower increases thereafter as indicated. In less acutely ill outpatients, dosage adjustments should be slower. Rapid dosage increases may cause patients to develop nausea and vomiting or mild neurologic toxicity such as drowsiness, dizziness, ataxia, clumsiness, or diplopia. Should such side effects occur, the dosage can be decreased temporarily and then increased again more slowly once they have passed. As noted previously, therapeutic blood levels for bipolar disorder have not been established. Some clinicians use the core range for epilepsy, 6–10 μg/ml, as a guide. Should blood levels be obtained to document a therapeutic trial or to establish an effective level for a given patient, trough levels are most meaningful and are conveniently drawn prior to the first morning dose. Given its elimination half-life, carbamazepine levels should be drawn no more frequently than 5 days after a dosage change. **Maintenance dosages** both for bipolar and epileptic patients average about 1000 mg/day, but the dosage range in routine clinical practice is large (200–1800 mg/day). The manufacturer recommends dosages no higher than 1600 mg/day.

Combinations with Lithium

Carbamazepine is used most often for bipolar patients who prove **resistant to treatment with lithium and/or valproic acid**. In many situations, therefore, the patient will already have a pharmacologic treatment for bipolar disorder that has been judged to be inadequate. In acute mania, carbamazepine can be either substituted for lithium or valproic acid or added to the initial drug. The primary danger of adding carbamazepine to lithium or valproic acid (and, in these situations, often also a neuroleptic and perhaps an antiparkinsonian and/or benzodiazepine) is risk of an acute combined central nervous system toxicity, for example, producing a confusional state. However, if the manic symptoms are severe enough to create pressure for rapid treatment, the physician may choose to add carbamazepine to the existing regimen because some patients respond only to combined therapy. If the patient improves, an attempt should be made to taper the lithium (or valproic acid) once the patient has stabilized. Some patients will worsen and require resumption of combined treatment. When such a combined regimen is undertaken, it is essential to minimize the dose of the antipsychotic drug (e.g., in the range of 8–10 mg of haloperidol or the equivalent). Unneeded anticholinergics and sedatives should also be decreased or omitted. In addition, it is important to have a clear idea of the patient's mental status and to consider the possibility of drug toxicity if the mental status worsens.

In the elderly and in patients whose mania is not so severe, it is preferable to substitute carbamazepine for lithium or valproic acid rather than add it. If the patient remains unresponsive, lithium or valproic acid can be added later. Whether a patient responds to carbamazepine alone or in combination with another mood stabilizer, it is good practice to taper and discontinue antipsychotic drugs once the acute episode has abated to minimize the risk of tardive dyskinesia.

Use in Pregnancy

Carbamazepine and other anticonvulsants cross the placenta. Fetal malformations caused by phenytoin (fetal hydantoin syndrome) have been well documented, and carbamazepine had been thought to be safer. However, a dissenting report (Jones et al., 1989) suggests that carbamazepine is also teratogenic. A prospective study of 35 children exposed to carbamazepine alone in utero found that 11% had craniofacial defects, 26% had fingernail hypoplasia, and 20% had developmental delay, similar to the abnormalities found with phenytoin. Pending further clarification, carbamazepine should be avoided if possible during pregnancy. Carbamazepine is secreted in breast milk at about 60% of the level found in the mother. Nursing children have been reported to become excessively drowsy. All anticonvulsants, including carbamazepine, are cleared more rapidly in pregnant females, leading to a fall in serum levels.

Side Effects and Toxicity

Although carbamazepine is associated with several serious toxicities (e.g., hepatitis, severe blood dyscrasias, and exfoliative dermatitis), these are fortunately extremely rare. In general, this drug is well tolerated, with fewer than 5% of patients discontinuing the

Table 5-4.   Side effects and toxicity of carbamazepine

Common dosage-related side effects
  Dizziness
  Ataxia
  Clumsiness
  Sedation
  Dysarthria
  Diplopia
  Nausea and gastrointestinal upset
  Reversible mild leukopenia
  Reversible mild increases in liver function tests
Less common dosage-related side effects
  Tremor
  Memory disturbance
  Confusional states (more common in elderly and in combination
     treatments with lithium or neuroleptics)
  Cardiac conduction delay
  Syndrome of inappropriate antidiuretic hormone (SIADH) secretion
Idiosyncratic toxicities
  Rash (including cases of exfoliation)
  Lenticular opacities
  Hepatitis
  Blood dyscrasias
     Aplastic anemia
     Leukopenia
     Thrombocytopenia

medication because of side effects. This compares favorably with the
older anticonvulsant, phenytoin. Most of carbamazepine's side
effects (Table 5-4) are neurologic or gastrointestinal symptoms due
to too rapid a dosage increase or excessively high serum levels.
These side effects can usually be avoided by increasing dosages
slowly and using the minimum effective dosage.

Neurologic Side Effects
Neurologic side effects are relatively common and may limit the
dosage that patients can tolerate. The most common are drowsiness,
vertigo, ataxia, diplopia, and blurred vision. When such side effects
occur, a decrease in dosage is indicated, but these side effects do not
represent a reason to stop therapy. When such side effects occur at
the initiation of therapy, a temporary dosage decrease with a slower
subsequent increase is often successful in permitting achievement of
a therapeutic dosage. Carbamazepine can also produce confusion,
the risk of which is higher when it is combined with antipsychotic
drugs or lithium. Risk factors for confusional states include old age
or underlying organic brain disease. In the absence of frank confusional states, carbamazepine appears to have little effect on memory
or other cognitive functions and is better than phenytoin in this
regard.

Hematologic Toxicity
Carbamazepine has both benign and severe hematologic toxicities.
It frequently is associated with clinically unimportant drops in
white blood cell counts and very rarely is associated with serious or
irreversible depression of red blood cells, white blood cells, or

platelets or a combination of these. Estimates of the rate of severe blood dyscrasias in the literature suggest an incidence of about 1 in 20,000 patients treated. As of 1982, there were 22 case reports of aplastic anemias (6 in the first month of treatment) and 17 cases of agranulocytosis.

Because carbamazepine often produces minor hematologic effects, it is important to have guidelines for identification of severe reactions, requiring discontinuation of the drug and close medical attention. Although there are no prospectively derived guidelines for psychiatric patients, Hart and Easton (1982) have made the following recommendations based on a review of the literature and clinical experience in neurologic patients:

1. Perform CBC and LFTs prior to treatment.
2. Consider patients with baseline abnormalities to be at high risk with closer follow-up monitoring.
3. During the first 2 months, check blood counts and LFTs every 2 weeks.
4. If no laboratory abnormalities appear and no symptoms of bone marrow suppression or hepatitis occur, obtain counts and LFTs every 3 months.
5. Stop the drug if white blood cell count drops below $3000/\mu l$ or neutrophil count drops below $1500/\mu l$, or in case of a threefold increase in LFTs.

Patients should be instructed to report fever, sore throat, pallor, unaccustomed weakness, petechiae, easy bruising, or bleeding. Concomitant use of lithium could potentially mask (but not reverse) carbamazepine-induced leukopenia. Thus, lithium should not be added to carbamazepine at times when a potentially serious drop in white blood cell count has occurred.

Cardiovascular Effects

Carbamazepine slows intracardiac conduction and may worsen preexisting cardiac conduction disease. Both sinus bradycardia and varying degrees of atrioventricular block have been reported. Carbamazepine is less dangerous in this regard than tricyclic antidepressants, but the existence of a high degree of heart block is a relative contraindication to its use. Other cardiovascular side effects listed by the manufacturer (e.g., congestive heart failure) are rare and may not be causally related to the drug.

Gastrointestinal Effects

Nausea and vomiting are relatively common dose-related side effects that do not necessitate termination of therapy. They are common at the start of therapy and, like dose-related neurologic side effects, can be minimized by increasing the dosage slowly. Mild, nonprogressive elevations of LFTs are also relatively common and require follow-up. The decision to continue the medication in the presence of mild LFT abnormalities must be individualized and should involve consultation with an internist or gastroenterologist.

Rarely, idiosyncratic, non-dose-related hepatitis may occur, usually in the first month of treatment. Patients generally manifest other signs of a hypersensitivity reaction, including fever and rash. Twenty cases were reported by 1985, of which about five were fatal. In the presence of such a reaction, carbamazepine should be permanently discontinued.

Dermatologic Effects

Rashes may develop in up to 3% of patients taking carbamazepine. Patients with urticaria and pruritic erythematous drug rashes should have the medication discontinued. Rarely, patients have developed Stevens-Johnson syndrome, which may be fatal.

Effects on Electrolytes

Carbamazepine has antidiuretic properties that can lead to **decreases in serum sodium.** These are usually clinically unimportant, but on rare occasions more severe hyponatremia may occur. Risk is highest in the elderly and in patients with a low serum sodium level at baseline. Appearance of new mental symptoms during carbamazepine treatment merits a check of serum electrolytes. Carbamazepine does not appear to be helpful in reversing lithium-induced polyuria.

Effects on Thyroid

Although long-term studies of patients on carbamazepine show decreases in free T_3 and T_4, reports of clinical hypothyroidism are anecdotal and rare. Carbamazepine is much less likely to produce significant effects on the thyroid than lithium, but hypothyroidism should be considered if a patient develops refractory depression.

Drug Interactions

Carbamazepine, like most anticonvulsants, may induce hepatic microsomal enzymes, resulting in increased metabolism of compounds that undergo hydroxylation or demethylation in the course of elimination. Significant drug interactions are listed in Table 5-5.

Overdose

Because of carbamazepine's slow absorption, peak levels in overdose may not be reached until the second or third day after the ingestion. Although it has a tricyclic structure, carbamazepine appears to be less dangerous in overdose than the tricyclic antidepressants. The major concerns in carbamazepine overdose are the development of high degrees of atrioventricular block (meriting cardiac monitoring) and stupor and coma, with risk of aspiration pneumonia. At higher doses, depression of respiration may occur, but it is usually relatively mild. Other symptoms and signs of overdose that have been reported include nystagmus, tremor, ballistic movements, mydriasis, ophthalmoplegia, orofacial dyskinesias, myoclonus, hypo- or hyperreflexia, rigidity, and seizures.

Management of carbamazepine overdoses is supportive. Because the drug is highly protein-bound, hemodialysis is of no benefit. Hemoperfusion confers uncertain benefit and does not appear to be indicated.

CLONAZEPAM

Clonazepam, a potent benzodiazepine, has been used primarily as an anticonvulsant, especially in the treatment of some childhood epilepsies. Uses of clonazepam in seizure disorders include

Absence (petit mal) seizures (ethosuximide preferred)
Atypical absence seizures
Infantile spasms

Table 5-5.   Drug interactions with carbamazepine

Diminishes Effects Of	Unpredictable Effects On	May Augment Effects Of	Carbamazepine Levels Decreased By	Carbamazepine Levels Increased By
Warfarin	Phenytoin	Digitalis (may induce or exacerbate bradycardia)	Phenobarbital	Erythromycin (marked increase)
Ethosuximide			Primidone	Isoniazid (marked increase)
Valproic Acid			Phenytoin	Propoxyphene
Tetracycline				Cimetidine
Haloperidol (probably)				SSRIs
Cyclic antidepressants (probably)				
Benzodiazepines including clonazepam				

Myoclonic seizures
Complex partial seizures (carbamazepine, phenytoin, and
  phenobarbital preferred)

Its use as an anticonvulsant has required high doses, with a corre-
spondingly high incidence of sedative side effects, development of
tolerance, reports of paradoxical excitement, and, rarely, induction
of psychotic-like symptoms. It has been shown to be effective at
lower dosages in the treatment of panic disorder with few side
effects. Like all benzodiazepines, it is a safe and effective sedative
when used as an adjunct to lithium and antipsychotic drugs in treating acute mania or other acute psychoses. A number of case reports
and small studies have suggested that clonazepam has specific antimanic (as opposed to general sedative) properties, but the evidence is
not strong and there have also been negative studies. Clonazepam is
fully discussed in Chapter 6.

BIBLIOGRAPHY

Valproic acid

Use in Bipolar Disorder

Bowden, C. L., Brugger, A. M., Swann, A. C., et al. Efficacy of divalproex
  vs lithium and placebo in the treatment of mania. *J.A.M.A.* 271 : 918,
  1994.
Calabrese, J. R., and Delucchi, G. A. Spectrum of efficacy of valproate in
  55 patients with rapid-cycling bipolar disorder. *Am. J. Psychiatry*
  147 : 431, 1990.
Calabrese, J. R., Markovitz, P., Kimmel, S. E., and Wagner, S. C. Spectrum of efficacy of valproate in 78 rapid-cycling bipolar patients.
  J. Clin. Psychopharmacol. 12 : 53S, 1992.
Freeman, T. W., Clothier, J. L., Pazzaglia, P., et al. A double-blind
  comparison of valproate and lithium in the treatment of acute mania.
  149 : 108, 1992.
Keck, P. E., McElroy, S. L., Vuckovic, A. V., and Friedman, L. M. Com-
  bined valproate and carbamazepine treatment of bipolar disorder.
  J. Neuropsychiatr. Clin. Neurosci. 4 : 319, 1992.
McElroy, S. L., Keck, P. E., Jr., Pope, H. G., Jr., and Hudson, J. I.
  Valproate in the treatment of rapid-cycling bipolar disorder. *J. Clin.
  Psychopharmacol.* 8 : 275, 1988.
Pope, H. G., Jr., McElroy, S. L., Keck, P. E., and Hudson, J. I. Valproate
  in the treatment of acute mania. *Arch. Gen. Psychiatry* 48 : 62, 1991.

Use in Other Psychiatric Disorders

McElroy, S. L., Keck, P. E., Jr., and Pope, H. G., Jr. Sodium valproate: Its
  use in primary psychiatric disorders. *J. Clin. Psychopharmacol.* 7 : 16,
  1987.

Side Effects and Toxicity

Dreifuss, F. E. Valproic acid hepatic fatalities: Revised table. *Neurology*
  39 : 1558, 1989.
Dreifuss, F. E., Langer, D. H., Moline, K. A., and Maxwell, J. E. Valproic
  acid hepatic fatalities II: U.S. experience since 1984. *Neurology*
  39 : 201, 1989.
Schnabel, R., Rainbeck, B., and Janssen, F. Fatal intoxication with
  sodium valproate. *Lancet* I : 221, 1984.
Smith, M. C. and Black, T. P. Convulsive disorders: toxicity of anticonvulsants. *Clin. Pharmacol.* 14 : 97, 1991.

Carbamazepine

Use in Bipolar Disorder

Frankenburg, F. R., Tohen, M., Cohen, B., and Lipinski, J. F., Jr. Long-term response to carbamazepine: A retrospective study. *J. Clin. Psychopharmacol.* 8 : 130, 1988.

Lusznat, R. M., Murphy, D. P., and Nunn, C. M. H. Carbamazepine vs. lithium in the treatment and prophylaxis of mania. *Br. J. Psychiatry* 153 : 198, 1986.

Placidi, G. F., Lenzi, A., Lazzerini, F., et al. The comparative efficacy and safety of carbamazepine versus lithium: A randomized, double-blind three-year trial in 83 patients. *J. Clin. Psychiatry* 47 : 490, 1986.

Post, R. M., Berrettini, W., Uhde, T. W., and Kellner, C. Selective response to the anticonvulsant carbamazepine in manic-depressive illness: A case study. *J. Clin. Psychopharmacol.* 4 : 178, 1984.

Post, R. M., Uhde, T. W., Ballenger, J. C., and Squillace, K. M. Prophylactic efficacy of carbamazepine in manic-depressive illness. *Am. J. Psychiatry* 140 : 1602, 1983.

Roy-Byrne, P. P., Joffe, R. T., Uhde, T. W., and Post, R. M. Approaches to the evaluation and treatment of rapid-cycling affective illness. *Br. J. Psychiatry* 145 : 543, 1984.

Schaffer, C. B., Mungas, D., and Rockwell, E. Successful treatment of psychotic depression with carbamazepine. *J. Clin. Psychopharmacol.* 5 : 233, 1985.

Small, J. G., Klapper, M. H., Milstein, V., et al. Carbamazepine compared with lithium in the treatment of mania. *Arch. Gen. Psychiatry* 48 : 915, 1991.

Stuppaeck, C., Barnas, C., Miller, C., et al. Carbamazepine in the prophylaxis of mood disorders. *J. Clin. Psychopharmacol.* 10 : 39, 1990.

Watkins, S. E., Callender, K., Thomas, D. R., et al. The effect of carbamazepine and lithium on remission from affective illness. *Br. J. Psychiatry* 150 : 180, 1987.

Use in Other Psychiatric Disorders

Gardner, D. L., and Cowdry, R. W. Positive effects of carbamazepine on behavioral dyscontrol in borderline personality disorder. *Am. J. Psychiatry* 143 : 519, 1986.

Malcolm, R., Ballenger, J. C., Sturgis, E. T., and Anton, R. Double-blind controlled trial comparing carbamazepine to oxazepam treatment of alcohol withdrawal. *Am. J. Psychiatry* 146 : 617, 1989.

Schweizer, E., Rickels, K., Case, W. G., and Greenblatt, D. J. Carbamazepine treatment in patients discontinuing long-term benzodiazepine therapy. *Arch. Gen. Psychiatry* 48 : 448, 1991.

Sramek, J., Herrera, J., Costa, J., et al. A carbamazepine trial in chronic, treatment-refractory schizophrenia. *Am. J. Psychiatry* 145 : 748, 1988.

Uhde, T. W., Stein, M. B., and Post, R. M. Lack of efficacy of carbamazepine in the treatment of panic disorder. *Am. J. Psychiatry* 145 : 1104, 1988.

Side Effects and Toxicity

Gardner, D. L., and Cowdry, R. W. Development of melancholia during carbamazepine treatment of borderline personality disorder. *J. Clin. Psychopharmacol.* 6 : 236, 1986.

Hart, R. G., and Easton, J. D. Carbamazepine and hematological monitoring. *Ann. Neurol.* 11 : 309, 1982.

Heh, C. W. C., Sramek, J., Herrera, J., and Costa, J. Exacerbation of psychosis after discontinuation of carbamazepine treatment. *Am. J. Psychiatry* 145 : 878, 1988.

Joffe, R. T., MacDonald, C., and Kutcher, S. P. Lack of differential cognitive effects of lithium and carbamazepine in bipolar affective disorder. *J. Clin. Psychopharmacol.* 8 : 425, 1988.

Joffe, R. T., Post, R. M., Roy-Byrne, P. P., and Uhde, T. W. Hematological effects of carbamazepine in patients with affective illness. *Am. J. Psychiatry* 142 : 1196, 1985.

Roy-Byrne, P. P., Joffe, R. T., Uhde, T. W., and Post, R. M. Carbamazepine and thyroid function in affectively ill patients. *Arch. Gen. Psychiatry* 41 : 1150, 1984.

Trimble, M. R., and Thompson, P. J. Anticonvulsant drugs, cognitive function, and behavior. *Epilepsia* 24(Suppl. 1) : S55, 1983.

Uhde, T. W., and Post, R. M. Effects of carbamazepine on serum electrolytes: Clinical and theoretical implications. *J. Clin. Psychopharmacol.* 3 : 103, 1983.

Zucker, P., Daum, F., and Cohen, M. Fatal carbamazepine hepatitis. *J. Pediatr.* 91 : 667, 1977.

Drug Interactions

Arana, G. W., Goff, D., Friedman, H., Ornsteen, M., et al. Does carbamazepine-induced lowering of haloperidol levels worsen psychotic symptoms? *Am. J. Psychiatry* 143 : 650, 1986.

Ketter, T. A., Post, R. M., and Worthington, K. Principles of clinically important drug interactions with carbamazepine: Parts I and II. *J. Clin Psychopharmacol.* 11 : 198, 1991; 11 : 306, 1991.

Shukla, S., Godwin, C. D., Long, L. E. B., and Miller, M. G. Lithium-carbamazepine neurotoxicity and risk factors. *Am. J. Psychiatry* 141 : 1604, 1984.

Use in Pregnancy

Jones, K. L., Johnson, K. A., and Adams, J. Pattern of malformations in children of women treated with carbamazepine during pregnancy. *N. Engl. J. Med.* 320 : 1661, 1989.

Rosa, F. W. Spina bifida in infants of women treated with carbamazepine during pregnancy. *N. Engl. J. Med.* 324 : 674, 1991.

6

Benzodiazepines and Other Anxiolytic Drugs

The benzodiazepine drugs have anxiolytic, sedative, anticonvulsant, and muscle relaxant properties, all of which are useful in clinical practice. A large number of benzodiazepines (Table 6-1) are currently available; recently a drug chemically unrelated to the benzodiazepines but with a similar receptor action (zolpidem) was introduced in the United States. Prior to the introduction of the benzodiazepines in 1960, a variety of compounds were employed to treat anxiety and insomnia. These included bromides early in the century, ethanol and structural analogs such as paraldehyde and chloral hydrate in the 1940s, followed by the barbiturates and propanediol drugs, including meprobamate, in the 1950s.

Benzodiazepines, like the older sedative-hypnotics, are central nervous system (CNS) depressants, with anxiolytic properties at relatively low doses and sedative-hypnotic effects (i.e., induction of drowsiness or sleep) at higher doses. The benzodiazepines have several clear advantages over the older drugs. Compared to barbiturates and similarly acting drugs, benzodiazepines have (1) a greater dose margin between anxiolysis and sedation, (2) less tendency to produce tolerance and dependence, (3) less abuse potential, and (4) a higher ratio of the median dose producing lethality to median effective dose (LD_{50}/ED_{50}). Indeed, the barbiturates and similarly acting drugs are quite dangerous in overdose—potentially causing coma, respiratory depression, and death. Since the introduction of benzodiazepines, the number of sleeping pill–related suicides and accidental deaths has decreased markedly. Given the advantages of benzodiazepines, the use of most of the older compounds (e.g., secobarbital, pentobarbital, meprobamate, glutethimide, or ethchlorvynol) for anxiolysis or sedation is irrational.

BENZODIAZEPINES

The effectiveness and relative safety of the benzodiazepines combined with the high frequency of complaints of anxiety and insomnia in medical practice have led to their extensive use. Despite a sharp decline in prescriptions for benzodiazepines over the last 15 years because of concerns about addiction and abuse, they are still widely prescribed. It is true that clinically significant dependence on benzodiazepines can occur even at therapeutic doses in the course of long-term use (> 6 months), and more rapidly with high-potency, short-acting benzodiazepines. Nonetheless it appears the risks of serious problems with dependence in the course of proper therapeutic use have been exaggerated; many patients continue to benefit from benzodiazepines with long-term use without obvious deleterious effects. Indeed, it is likely that, at present, excessive fears of "addicting" patients may be contributing to withholding potentially effective therapy from many anxious patients. On the other hand, the potential for inducing dependence, especially with some of the more potent short-acting drugs such as alprazolam and lorazepam, must be taken seriously by physicians. In general, benzodiazepines should neither be withheld because of prejudice nor

Table 6-1. Available anxiolytic and hypnotic preparations

Available Preparations	Regular Oral Dosage Forms (mg)	Slow-Release Forms (mg)	Parenteral Forms (mg)
Alprazolam (Xanax)[a]	0.25, 0.5, 1.0, 2.0 (Tab)		
Buspirone (BuSpar)[c]	5, 10 (Tab)		
Chlordiazepoxide[b] Librium and others	5, 10, 25 (Tab) 5, 10, 25 (Cap)		100 mg/2 ml (Amp)
Clonazepam (Klonopin)	0.5, 1.0, 2.0 (Tab)		
Clorazepate (Tranxene) and generics	3.75, 7.5, 15.0 (Tab) 3.75, 7.5 (Cap)	11.25, 22.5	
Diazepam (Valium and generics)	2, 5, 10 (Tab)	15	10 mg/2 ml (Amp or Syr) 50 mg/10 ml (Vial)
Estazolam (ProSom)	1, 2 (Tab)		
Flurazepam (Dalmane) and generics	15, 30 (Cap)		
Lorazepam (Ativan)[a] and generics	0.5, 1.0, 2.0 (Tab)		20 mg/10 ml, 40 mg/10 ml (Vial) 2 mg/ml, 4 mg/ml (Syr)
Midazolam (Versed)			1 mg/ml 5 mg/ml (Vial)

Oxazepam (Serax and generics)	15 (Tab)
	10, 15, 30 (Cap)
Quazepam (Doral)	7.5, 15.0 (Tab)
Temazepam (Restoril) and generics	7.5, 15.0, 30.0 (Cap)
Triazolam (Halcion)	0.125, 0.25 (Tab)
Zolpidem (Ambien)[c]	5, 10 (Tab)

[a]Tablets can be taken sublingually for use requiring more rapid onset of action.
[b]Available with clidinium bromide (Librax, Clipoxide) and amitriptyline (Limbitrol).
Preparation forms available: tablets (Tab); capsules (Cap); vials (Vial); ampules (Amp); prefilled syringes (Syr).
[c]Nonbenzodiazepines.

prescribed indiscriminately without a careful diagnostic evaluation. Rational use of benzodiazepines is based on

1. Presence of a benzodiazepine-responsive syndrome
2. Use of appropriate nonpharmacologic therapies when indicated
3. Assessment of the approximate duration of treatment (e.g., avoiding open-ended treatment of insomnia, but recognizing that many anxiety disorders may require long-term therapy)
4. Consideration of the risk-benefit factors associated with benzodiazepine treatment for individual patients (e.g., benzodiazepines should be avoided in patients with a history of alcohol or drug abuse unless there is a very compelling indication, no good alternative, and close follow-up)
5. Adjustment of dosage to optimize therapeutic effects and minimize side effects (e.g., drowsiness)
6. Monitoring for abuse (unsupervised dose acceleration or diversion to other individuals)
7. Slowly tapering the drug after an appropriate trial to determine need for any further treatment
8. Reconsideration of diagnosis if the patient is poorly responsive, if medication is needed longer, or if higher doses than originally estimated are needed

Chemistry

The benzodiazepines are a group of closely related compounds whose structures are depicted in Fig. 6-1. The name *benzodiazepine* is derived from the fact that the structures are composed of a benzene ring fused to a seven-member diazepine ring. A chemically unrelated compound, zolpidem, has recently been introduced in the United States, but it acts on the same family of receptors as the benzodiazepines.

Pharmacology

Dependence

Clinically, the major pharmacologic problem with benzodiazepines is their tendency to cause dependence, that is, a risk of significant discontinuation symptoms, especially with long-term use. Long-term benzodiazepine use occurs in medical settings because both panic disorder and generalized anxiety disorder often run chronic courses. Discontinuation symptoms may pose a serious clinical problem in some patients, causing distress or inability to discontinue treatment. However, it is the widespread confusion of **pharmacologic dependence** with **drug addiction** that has most complicated the clinical use of benzodiazepines.

Dependence means that on drug cessation, an individual experiences pathologic symptoms and signs. In the past, it was often taught that physical dependence, as manifested by physical withdrawal symptoms (e.g., tremor or elevated blood pressure) appearing with drug cessation, was the key indicator of drug addiction. This concept has now appropriately been abandoned. Some highly addictive drugs, such as cocaine, do not produce a physical withdrawal syndrome. Moreover, many medically useful drugs, such as the antihypertensive drugs clonidine and propranolol, may produce physical dependence (e.g., rebound hypertension or angina on cessation) without producing addictive behaviors. Rather than basing the concept of addiction on physical dependence, addiction is now under-

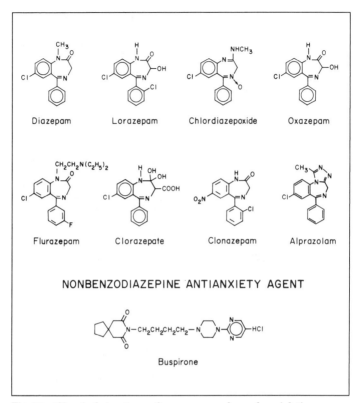

Fig. 6-1.   Chemical structures of some commonly used anxiolytics.

stood as a cluster of cognitive, affective, behavioral, and physiologic signs that indicate compulsive use of a substance and inability to control intake despite negative consequences such as medical illness, failure in life roles, and marked interpersonal difficulties.

DSM-IV does not use the term *addiction* because it has collected a variety of imprecise and pejorative meanings. However, the DSM-III and DSM-IV use of *drug dependence* to signify addiction raises the specter of serious misunderstandings among both physicians and patients for the medical use of benzodiazepines (and also of narcotic analgesics). The terminal cancer patient with severe pain is likely to become both physically and psychologically dependent on prescribed opiate analgesics but is not an "addict"; that is, the person has not "lost control" over the drug and is not engaged in maladaptive compulsive drug-seeking behaviors. Moreover, were the pain to stop, the individual would not experience drug craving. Similarly, the patient with panic disorder may also become dependent on prescribed benzodiazepines; that is, the patient might have rebound anxiety and even withdrawal symptoms (e.g., tachycardia) with discontinuation but is not in any way an addict. The confusion of dependence and addiction can lead to unnecessary shame for patients and, more importantly, to undermedication even when the drug is indicated. While it is true that polydrug abusers may misuse benzodiazepines and become addicted to them in the true sense of the term, benzodiazepines are intrinsically far less addictive than opiates, cocaine, alcohol, barbiturates, or nicotine. Restrictive prescribing laws (e.g., as are currently in force in New York) effectively decrease benzodiazepine prescriptions but may lead to increased prescription of more dangerous and less effective drugs such as meprobamate, methyprylon, and barbiturates. Such laws also put stigma and other obstacles in the way of appropriate anxiolytic therapies.

Choosing a Benzodiazepine

All benzodiazepines and likely the nonbenzodiazepine zolpidem appear to have essentially the same mechanism of action and side effects that are similar. Of all of the drugs used in psychiatry, benzodiazepines are the class in which pharmacokinetic considerations play the greatest role in selecting a drug for a particular situation. The dosage forms, rate of onset of action, duration of action, and tendency to accumulate in the body vary considerably and can influence both side effects and the overall success of the treatment. The other major consideration in choosing a benzodiazepine drug is potency; only the most potent agents have general utility in the treatment of panic disorder and certain epilepsies, but high potency may increase the risk of dependence.

Route of Administration

ORAL USE. Most benzodiazepines are well absorbed when given orally on an empty stomach; many achieve peak plasma levels within 1–3 hours, although there is a wide range among the benzodiazepine drugs (Table 6-2). Antacids seriously interfere with benzodiazepine absorption; thus, benzodiazepines should be taken well ahead of any antacid dose.

The rate of onset of action after an orally administered benzodiazepine (Table 6-2) may be an important variable in choosing a drug. For example, rapid onset is important when emergency sedation is required or for the individual who has trouble falling asleep. On the other hand, a more slowly acting drug might be prescribed when insomnia occurs later in the night. Drugs with a rapid onset achieve higher peak levels than equivalent doses of drugs with slow onset, whose peaks are spread over time (Fig. 6-2). The psychotropic effects of drugs with rapid onset, such as diazepam or clorazepate, are often distinctly felt by patients both because of the rapid change in drug level and because the peak level is high. Patients may experience rapidly acting drugs as positively or negatively reinforcing; some patients expect to feel the onset of action of a dose, interpreting this as therapeutic. Others have a dysphoric response, complaining of sedation or loss of control. This latter group of patients often do better on a drug with a slow onset of action. It is worth asking about such reactions in follow-up. Patients who are drug abusers may interpret peak effects as a desirable "high"; thus, patients with drug abuse histories might be given an agent with slow onset (e.g., oxazepam), if given a benzodiazepine at all.

The available benzodiazepines differ markedly in the rate of onset of their therapeutic effect (see Table 6-2), offering a wide choice of drugs to fit the patient's needs. Diazepam, a rapidly absorbed compound, usually achieves peak levels within 1 hour after an oral dose.

Table 6-2.   Data on available benzodiazepines

Available Preparations	Oral Dosage Equivalency (mg)	Onset After Oral Dose	Distribution Half-life	Elimination Half-life (hr)[a]
Alprazolam (Xanax)	0.5	Intermediate	Intermediate	6–20
Chlordiazepoxide (Librium and generics)	10.0	Intermediate	Slow	30–100
Clonazepam (Klonopin)	0.25	Intermediate	Intermediate	18–50
Clorazepate[b] (Tranxene)	7.5	Rapid	Rapid	30–100
Diazepam (Valium and generics)	5.0	Rapid	Rapid	30–100
Estazolam (ProSom)	2.0	Intermediate	Intermediate	10–24
Flurazepam (Dalmane)	30.0	Rapid-intermediate	Rapid	50–160
Lorazepam (Ativan and generics)	1.0	Intermediate	Intermediate	10–20
Midazolam (Versed)	—	Intermediate	Rapid	2–3
Oxazepam (Serax)	15.0	Intermediate-slow	Intermediate	8–12
Quazepam (Doral)	15.0	Rapid-intermediate	Intermediate	50–160
Temazepam (Restoril)	30.0	Intermediate	Rapid	8–20
Triazolam (Halcion)	0.25	Intermediate	Rapid	1.5–5

[a]The elimination half-life represents the total for all active metabolites; the elderly tend to have the longer half-lives in the range reported. Chlordiazepoxide, clorazepate, and diazepam have desmethyldiazepam as a long-lived active metabolite. Flurazepam and quazepam share N-desalkylflurazepam as a long-lived active metabolite. With chronic dosing, these active metabolites represent most of the pharmacodynamic effect of these drugs.

[b]Clorazepate is an inactive prodrug for desmethyldiazepam, which is the active compound in the blood.

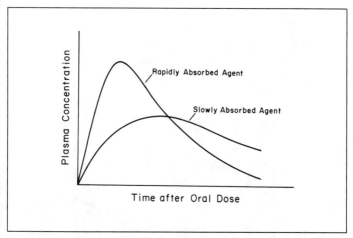

Fig. 6-2. Comparison of peak levels achieved related to rate of absorption. The curves could represent a comparison of levels for a single drug given rapidly versus slowly IV. The curves could also represent peak levels for equivalent doses of two similar drugs with different rates of absorption. The more rapidly absorbed drug achieves a higher peak level.

SUBLINGUAL USE. Several benzodiazepines (nongeneric forms of lorazepam, alprazolam, and triazolam) are compounded to permit either sublingual or oral administration. The time to peak levels appears to be only slightly faster by the sublingual route and may not represent a clinically significant difference from the oral route. However, the sublingual route may be a useful alternative for patients who cannot swallow pills or for patients who have a full stomach, which would delay oral absorption. When used sublingually, tablets should be placed under the tongue and allowed to dissolve passively. Dry mouth may lead to a lack of dissolution of the tablet. Depending on how they are compounded, generic forms may not be absorbed sublingually.

INTRAMUSCULAR USE. Absorption of benzodiazepines after intramuscular administration varies according to drug and site of administration. Drugs are better absorbed from better perfused muscle groups. Specifically, it appears that lorazepam, midazolam, and perhaps diazepam are well absorbed if given in the deltoid muscle, a site that is preferable to the vastus lateralis or gluteus maximus. Chlordiazepoxide is not reliably absorbed when administered intramuscularly, regardless of site; therefore, chlordiazepoxide should not be administered by this route.

INTRAVENOUS USE. Benzodiazepines are commonly administered intravenously for preoperative sedation and in treating seizures. In psychiatric practice, benzodiazepines are used intravenously only in serious emergency situations. Intravenous diazepam, lorazepam, or midazolam is useful for the control of antipsychotic-induced laryngeal dystonia if anticholinergics fail (see Chap. 2) and for emergency sedation in extremely agitated or delirious states. Of these three drugs, lorazepam has the longest-lasting effects after a single intra-

Table 6-3.   Clinical relevance of pharmacokinetics of benzodiazepines

Situations in which single-dose kinetics are important
  Treatment of insomnia (one night)
  Sleep during travel across time zones
  Emergency treatment of acute anxiety or agitation
  Emergency sedation of patients with acute psychosis
  Status epilepticus
  Preoperative sedation
  Induction of anesthesia

Situations in which multiple-dose kinetics are important
  Long-term treatment of anxiety
  Nightly treatment of insomnia (consecutive nights)
  Intermediate-term adjunctive use with antidepressants
  Long-term treatment of neuroleptic-induced akathisia

venous dose because it is less quickly and extensively distributed into lipid stores than diazepam, which is a critical parameter after a single emergency dose (see Duration of Effect). Midazolam has an extremely short elimination half-life.

Whenever benzodiazepines are given intravenously, they should be given slowly (over a minute or two) instead of by rapid push; over-rapid administration will produce very high blood levels, resulting in excessive risk of respiratory arrest (see Fig. 6-2). Benzodiazepines should only be given intravenously if personnel are trained and equipped to deal with possible respiratory arrest.

Duration of Effect

For benzodiazepines, simple half-life data are potentially misleading regarding duration of clinical effect. Clinical efficacy depends on the presence of at least a minimum effective concentration in the blood, which is reflected by levels in well-perfused tissues such as those in the brain. After a single dose, the levels may fall to ineffective concentrations either (1) by being distributed into peripheral tissues, such as fat (referred to as alpha phase, with a time course described by the distribution half-life), or (2) by metabolic inactivation or elimination from the body altogether (referred to as beta phase, with a time course described by the elimination half-life).

The volume of distribution represents the "size" of the pool of tissues into which the drug may be drawn; this is determined by the drug's lipid solubility and tissue-binding properties. With repeated drug dosing, its "volume of distribution" becomes saturated, and the elimination half-life becomes the more important parameter in describing its behavior. Benzodiazepines differ markedly in their half-lives of distribution and elimination, producing varying clinical effects.

These pharmacokinetic considerations have clear clinical relevance in the use of benzodiazepines (Table 6-3). When acute doses of benzodiazepines are to be used (e.g., in emergency situations), the rates of absorption and distribution are critical (the latter because benzodiazepines lose their biologic effect by redistribution into the tissues much more rapidly than by elimination from the body). With repeated dosing, on the other hand, distribution is complete, and the elimination half-life, which determines the steady state levels of the drug, becomes the important factor.

Table 6-4. Clinical importance of long versus short half-life of elimination with repeat dosing

Long Half-life		Short Half-life	
Advantages	*Disadvantages*	*Advantages*	*Disadvantages*
Less frequent dosing	Accumulation (problem in the elderly)	No accumulation	More frequent dosing
Lack of interdose rebound anxiety or insomnia	Greater risk of next-day sedation after use for insomnia	Less daytime drowsiness after repeated nightly use as hypnotic	Rebound insomnia (especially after use of high-potency compounds on several consecutive nights)
Withdrawal problems less severe			Interdose rebound anxiety and early morning anxiety (with high-potency compounds)

These points can be demonstrated in the clinical use of two commonly employed drugs, diazepam and lorazepam. The distribution half-life (alpha phase) for oral diazepam is 2.5 hours, whereas the elimination half-life (beta phase) is more than 30 hours. Desmethyldiazepam, diazepam's major active metabolite, extends the overall elimination half-life to 60–100 hours (up to 200 hours in the elderly). This means that a single dose of diazepam will be active for a relatively short period of time based on the rapid distribution of the drug, whereas with repeated administration, elimination half-life becomes the important parameter to consider, making diazepam a very long-acting drug (i.e., one that will accumulate in the body to high levels). Conversely, despite the relatively short elimination half-life of lorazepam (10 hours) and its lack of active metabolites, it has a smaller volume of distribution than diazepam and therefore a longer action when given as a single dose. Thus, for a single emergency dose (e.g., for acute sedation or an intravenous dose for status epilepticus), lorazepam would have a significantly longer-lasting clinical effect than diazepam and might therefore be preferable. With repeated dosing, however, lorazepam is shorter acting than diazepam and is therefore unlikely to build up to high levels, as diazepam does (Table 6-4).

Another important clinical issue related to duration of effect is relevant to the use of the high-potency, short-acting benzodiazepines, alprazolam, triazolam, and midazolam, and to a lesser extent lorazepam. Such drugs pose a unique clinical problem because their high potency may make them more liable to cause dependence and their rapid termination of effect unmasks any dependence that develops. Patients may therefore experience rebound symptoms between scheduled doses. For example, some patients treated with alprazolam for panic disorder develop severe rebound anxiety between doses, unless their dose frequency is increased to 4–5 doses/day. Patients treated with triazolam for insomnia may develop rebound symptoms within one dose, as manifested by early morning awakening or anxiety. Such problems can be dealt with by switching to longer-acting drugs when indicated (e.g., replacing alprazolam with clonazepam for panic anxiety [method described under Tolerance and Discontinuation Symptoms]) or by replacing triazolam with temazepam or flurazepam for insomnia.

Metabolism

Except for lorazepam, oxazepam, and temazepam, the commonly used benzodiazepines are metabolized by hepatic microsomal enzymes to form demethylated, hydroxylated, and other oxidized products that are pharmacologically active. These active metabolites are, in turn, conjugated with glucuronic acid; the resulting glucuronides are inactive, and because they are more water-soluble than the parent compounds, they are readily excreted in the urine. Major metabolic pathways for benzodiazepines are shown in Figure 6-3.

Some of the active metabolites of benzodiazepines, such as desmethyldiazepam and desalkylflurazepam, have extremely long half-lives and with repeat dosing may represent most of the pharmacologically active compound in serum. In contrast, under normal circumstances (e.g., excluding cirrhosis) the active metabolic products of alprazolam, triazolam, and midazolam are of little clinical importance.

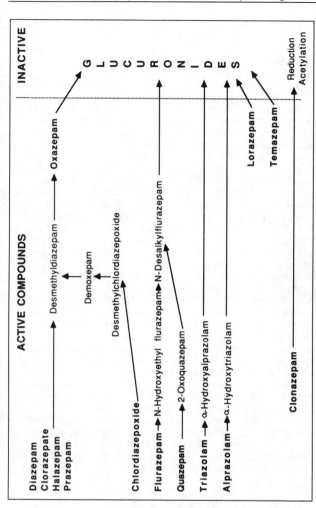

Fig. 6-3. Metabolic pathways of major benzodiazepines. Compounds marketed in the United States are shown in boldface type. All compounds to the left of the dotted line are active except clorazepate, which is a prodrug for desmethyldiazepam.

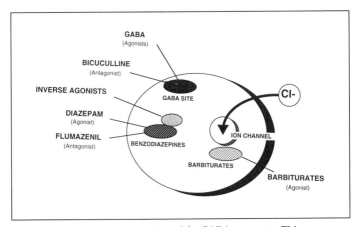

Fig. 6-4.   Schematic representation of the GABA$_A$ receptor. This diagram illustrates three of the major binding sites on the GABA$_A$ receptor and the chloride channel, but does not represent the actual subunit structure of the receptor. The chloride channel opens when two molecules of GABA bind to their site on the receptor. The proconvulsant compound bicuculline blocks the binding of GABA to its site. The benzodiazepine and barbiturate binding sites are physically separate from the GABA site and from each other. Compounds such as flumazenil, with no intrinsic activity, compete with benzodiazepines such as diazepam for binding and thus serve as benzodiazepine antagonists.

Lorazepam, oxazepam, and temazepam are metabolized only by conjugation with glucuronic acid with no intermediate steps, and they have no active metabolites. Unlike the pathways involved in the initial metabolism of other benzodiazepines, glucuronidation is less affected by aging and liver disease; thus, if benzodiazepines are to be used in elderly patients or those with cirrhosis, lorazepam and oxazepam are the drugs of choice. In cirrhosis, the elimination of benzodiazepines metabolized by oxidation and demethylation may be reduced by as much as fivefold; thus, routine doses could lead to serious toxicity. In cirrhosis, even alprazolam, triazolam, and midazolam may accumulate to dangerous levels.

Mechanism of Action

Acting through its GABA$_A$ receptor, the amino acid neurotransmitter gamma-aminobutyric acid (GABA) is the major inhibitory neurotransmitter in the brain. GABA$_A$ receptors are ligand-gated channels, meaning that the neurotransmitter-binding site and an effector ion channel are part of the same macromolecular complex. Because GABA$_A$ receptor channels selectively admit the anion chloride into neurons, activation of GABA$_A$ receptors hyperpolarizes neurons and thus is inhibitory. Benzodiazepines produce their effects by binding to a specific site on the GABA$_A$ receptor.

The pharmacology of GABA$_A$ receptors is complex; GABA$_A$ receptors are the primary site of action not only of benzodiazepines but also of barbiturates and of some of the intoxicating effects of ethanol. The multiple drug and neurotransmitter-binding sites associated with the GABA$_A$ receptor are schematized in Figure 6-4.

Benzodiazepines and barbiturates act at separate binding sites on the receptor to potentiate the inhibitory action of GABA. They do so by allosterically regulating the receptor (changing its conformation) so that it has a greater affinity for GABA. In addition, each drug increases the affinity of the receptor for the other. Ethanol also allosterically modifies the receptor so that it has increased affinity for GABA and the other drugs. It does so not by binding to the receptor itself, but by altering the membrane environment of the receptor. At higher doses, barbiturates and ethanol, but not benzodiazepines, can also open the chloride channel within the receptor independent of GABA. The fact that benzodiazepines, barbiturates, and ethanol all have related actions on a common receptor explains their pharmacologic synergy (and therefore the dangers of combined overdose) and their cross-tolerance. Their cross-tolerance is exploited in detoxification of alcoholics with benzodiazepines.

It has recently become clear that $GABA_A$ receptors are constructed of multiple subunits. Active $GABA_A$ receptors appear to contain two alpha subunits, two beta subunits, and a gamma or delta subunit. Only those $GABA_A$ receptors that contain gamma subunits can interact with benzodiazepines. Multiple different alpha, beta, and gamma subunits have been discovered. The actual diversity of $GABA_A$ receptors in the brain (i.e., how the different types of subunits are mixed and matched) is only now being established and related to pharmacologic data. The diversity of $GABA_A$ receptors raises the possibility of far more selective benzodiazepine-like drugs in the future, perhaps drugs that are anxiolytic with less sedative effects or even with less tendency to produce dependence.

Although it is known that benzodiazepines and zolpidem produce their primary actions by allosterically regulating $GABA_A$ receptors, it is not entirely clear how they function as anxiolytics. Specifically, given the ubiquity of $GABA_A$ receptors in the brain, it is not clear how benzodiazepines achieve specificity as anxiolytics when used at therapeutic doses. It must be asked which of the many GABAergic synapses in the brain are actually relevant to benzodiazepine-induced anxiolysis and what are their normal functions. Based on animal models, it is believed that the anxiolytic properties of benzodiazepines reflect their inhibitory actions on neurons within the limbic system, including the amygdala and on serotonergic (5-HT) and noradrenergic neurons within the brainstem. In contrast, the anticonvulsant actions of benzodiazepines may represent action on cortical neurons.

ZOLPIDEM

Zolpidem appears to interact with a smaller subset of $GABA_A$ than the benzodiazepines. It is therefore pharmacologically cross-reactive with the benzodiazepines to a degree. Zolpidem is effective for short-term treatment of insomnia. It lacks significant anxiolytic, muscle relaxant, or anticonvulsant effects. It is rapidly and completely absorbed from the gastrointestinal tract, reaching peak serum levels in 1–2 hours. Its absorption is delayed by food. Zolpidem is metabolized by the liver, with a short elimination half-life of 2.5 hours. The half-life is prolonged in the elderly and in patients with liver disease. The major side effects of zolpidem are nausea, vomiting, diarrhea, headache, and dizziness. Like benzodiazepines, zolpidem may produce anterograde amnesia and rebound insomnia, especially at higher doses. Its safety in overdose and its liability for abuse remain to be established.

BUSPIRONE

Buspirone is a nonbenzodiazepine anxiolytic that has been approved for treatment of generalized anxiety disorder. It is a member of a chemical group called the azaspirodecanediones, which have not previously been used in psychopharmacology. Buspirone has no direct effects on $GABA_A$ receptors; it has no pharmacologic cross-reactivity with benzodiazepines or barbiturates, and it lacks the sedative, anticonvulsant, and muscle relaxant effects of benzodiazepines. A major advantage of buspirone is that it does not appear to produce dependence, and it seems to have little or no abuse potential.

Buspirone is believed to exert its anxiolytic effect by acting as a partial agonist at $5\text{-}HT_{1a}$ receptors. Serotonin is thought to act as an anxiogenic neurotransmitter in limbic structures. Since $5\text{-}HT_{1a}$ receptors are autoreceptors, their activation by buspirone decreases serotonin turnover, so according to the theory, buspirone is anxiolytic. However, investigations of the role of serotonin in anxiety are in their early stages. Of interest, buspirone has an active metabolite 1-phenyl-piperazine (1-PP) that acts via alpha$_2$-adrenergic receptors to increase the rate of firing of locus ceruleus neurons. Whether this stimulation of adrenergic systems, which would be unwanted in anxiety disorders, limits the efficacy of buspirone is unclear.

Buspirone is 100% absorbed from the human gastrointestinal tract but undergoes extensive first-pass metabolism by the liver so that only 4% may be bioavailable. Buspirone is metabolized by the liver; the half-life of the parent compound is 2–11 hours.

When used to treat generalized anxiety disorder, buspirone has been found to be as effective as standard benzodiazepine treatments in some but not all studies. Buspirone is most often ineffective as a sole treatment for panic disorder. It appears that patients with generalized anxiety disorder who have taken benzodiazepines within 4 weeks prior to taking buspirone may be less likely to benefit from buspirone. Unlike benzodiazepines, buspirone is effective only when taken regularly. It takes 1–2 weeks to show its initial effects, and maximal effectiveness may be reached only after 4–6 weeks. This must be clearly explained to patients who are accustomed to using benzodiazepines. Because of this time course of effectiveness, buspirone is not useful in emergencies or when rapid onset of anxiolysis is required. The initial dosage of buspirone is 5 mg tid; in most trials, 20–30 mg/day in 3 divided doses has been effective, but a total dosage of up to 60 mg/day has been used.

Due to its lack of cross-reactivity with benzodiazepines, buspirone cannot prevent benzodiazepine withdrawal symptoms. Therefore, when switching patients from a benzodiazepine to buspirone, the benzodiazepine must be slowly tapered as if no new drug were being introduced. If buspirone is started before the taper has concluded (which should be safe), it is important not to confuse benzodiazepine withdrawal or rebound symptoms with buspirone side effects.

Buspirone does not cause sedation; it *may* occasionally produce restlessness. It does not appear to impair psychomotor performance.

Headache, gastrointestinal distress, dizziness, and paresthesia have been reported but are infrequent. There is little experience with overdose, but buspirone does not appear to be highly toxic.

Buspirone has been somewhat disappointing in general clinical use in that a smaller percentage of anxious patients benefit from buspirone than from benzodiazepines. Whether this reflects inappropriate expectations and use on the part of both physicians and patients who are accustomed to the rapid effects of benzodiazepines remains to be established. For patients who respond to buspirone, it has the marked advantages of being free of sedation and lacking any prominent discontinuation symptomatology.

INDICATIONS FOR BENZODIAZEPINES, ZOLPIDEM, AND BUSPIRONE

Although benzodiazepines are marketed for different indications, such as flurazepam, temazepam, and triazolam for insomnia, or diazepam for anxiety, muscle relaxation, and preoperative sedation, it is likely that all of the drugs in this class share most of their therapeutic properties. The differences in approved indications largely reflect selective research and marketing decisions rather than rational therapeutics. In other words, diazepam works well for insomnia, and flurazepam would serve as an anxiolytic. In most cases, drug choice is best made on the basis of pharmacokinetic differences and potency (as discussed previously). Potency is particularly important in the treatment of panic attacks, in which high-potency benzodiazepines (e.g., alprazolam and clonazepam) have clear therapeutic advantages. The high-potency and long half-life of clonazepam make it uniquely valuable in the treatment of certain epilepsies. The nonbenzodiazepine buspirone may be effective for some patients with generalized anxiety, but not for panic disorder. In addition to questions about its general efficacy, its major disadvantage is slow onset of effect.

Anxiety

Anxiety is a ubiquitous human emotion. Most instances of anxiety do not call for medical treatment. However, anxiety can become severe enough that it impairs the ability of the individual to act adaptively; in such circumstances, treatment should be considered. Anxiety may be (1) a normal response to stressful life events, (2) a symptom of an anxiety disorder, (3) a symptom of another psychiatric disorder such as depression, or (4) a symptom of a medical illness, such as thyrotoxicosis.

Situational or Stress-Related Anxiety

This is usually self-limited and rarely calls for medical treatment. When patients complain of anxiety due to a specific life stress, the questions to address include the following:

1. Is the anxiety harmful to the individual? In many situations anxiety may be helpful in terms of ability to perform, but in other situations anxiety can lead to maladaptive behavior or extreme dysphoria. In such situations, treatment is indicated.
2. Would psychological treatment be effective and acceptable to the patient?

3. What are the risks of short-term benzodiazepine treatment? Specifically, the physician must consider side effects, the acceptability of pharmacologic treatment to the individual, possible dependency, and possible interactions with underlying medical disorders.

If drug treatment is indicated, a low-potency, long-acting benzodiazepine might be prescribed. Such compounds have the lowest risk of causing dependence and subsequent withdrawal symptoms. A typical regimen might be diazepam, 5 mg tid or the equivalent. Doses may be increased as needed, but the equivalent of 30 mg of diazepam or less should suffice for almost all cases of situational anxiety. The duration of treatment should be limited, guided by the time course of the stressor that precipitated the anxiety.

Benzodiazepines can also be useful for the symptomatic treatment of transient anxiety, fear, or tension associated with medical illnesses (e.g., post–myocardial infarction) and surgical illnesses (e.g., for pre- or postoperative anxiety). The dosage is similar to that for other situational anxieties, usually less than the equivalent of 30 mg/day of diazepam. In the elderly or in patients with compromised hepatic function, lorazepam or oxazepam is a better choice because it will not accumulate; in such patients, lower doses are prudent.

Social Phobia and Performance Anxiety

Social phobia, as defined by DSM-IV, represents persistent fears of one or more social situations in which the person is exposed to possible scrutiny by others and fears humiliation. Perhaps the best known example is stage fright, in which an individual is unable to speak or perform in public. Other social phobias include being unable to speak in class or in social situations. If severe, social phobia can cause both social and occupational impairment because of avoidance of phobic situations.

In **stage fright**, the major troublesome symptoms are autonomic, such as pounding heart, dry mouth, and tremor. Because benzodiazepines may adversely affect mental acuity, the treatment of choice is usually a beta-adrenergic blocker, such as propranolol, which is likely to have fewer mental side effects (see Chap. 7). Clinical reports have also suggested efficacy of the longer-acting beta-adrenergic blocker atenolol for discrete social phobias, but not for the generalized form of the disorder. Cognitive and behavior therapies, whether offered in individual or group settings, are frequently effective in diminishing distress and avoidance and may be combined with pharmacotherapies.

For other types of social phobia, there is evidence that benzodiazepines may be helpful. If the phobic situation is encountered rarely, as-needed use of a benzodiazepine (e.g., diazepam, 5 mg) may be helpful. For individuals whose social phobia causes pervasive avoidance of interpersonal interactions, prescription of a regular dose of a benzodiazepine may be helpful, especially if combined with cognitive/behavior therapies. Anecdotal reports support the use of alprazolam and clonazepam for social phobia as with panic disorder, and controlled trial data indicate superiority of clonazepam over placebo. There is also controlled trial evidence for efficacy of the monoamine oxidase inhibitors (MAOIs), phenelzine and tranylcypromine in social phobia (see Chap. 3).

Generalized Anxiety Disorder

Generalized anxiety disorder (GAD) is a primary anxiety disorder characterized by unrealistic and excessive ongoing worry (> 6 months) accompanied by specific anxiety symptoms such as motor tension, autonomic hyperactivity, or excessive vigilance. Whether GAD represents a valid diagnostic entity or a heterogeneous group of patients remains to be seen, but the diagnosis may be clinically useful because it provides criteria for identifying a group of patients who have similar treatment needs and whose management poses similar difficulties.

It is important to be careful about the diagnosis of GAD because generalized anxiety symptoms are often features of other major psychiatric disorders, medical disorders, or medications or drugs (secondary anxiety). Anxiety symptoms often accompany depression, psychoses, obsessive-compulsive disorder, and other psychiatric disorders. They also may be the manifestation of medical illnesses such as angina, congestive heart failure, arrhythmias, asthma and other obstructive pulmonary diseases, and hyperthyroidism, or they may result from overuse of aminophylline, thyroid supplements, caffeine, or over-the-counter decongestants or appetite suppressants. Secondary anxiety may also be the result of withdrawal from alcohol or other CNS depressants. Secondary anxiety is best approached by treatment of the underlying disorder, although in many situations, short-term use of adjunctive benzodiazepines may be helpful. In some cases (e.g., in certain respiratory disorders), however, a benzodiazepine may prove harmful.

There is a paucity of research on the treatment of GAD. Benzodiazepines are usually helpful but are best combined with a non-pharmacologic treatment (e.g., cognitive or behavior therapy). Generally, low-potency, long-acting benzodiazepines are safe and effective. High-potency, short-acting compounds, such as alprazolam, carry too high a risk of dependence and interdose rebound symptoms to be considered first-line therapies for GAD. Typically, dosages of 15–30 mg/day of diazepam or the equivalent are effective, but occasional patients have required the equivalent of 40–60 mg/day of diazepam. Some patients with generalized anxiety improve with short-term (2–6 weeks) treatment, but the majority will have recurrences if treatment is stopped at that time. Long-term treatment (> 6 months) appears to be safe and effective for many patients; nonetheless, it is worth trying to taper the medication periodically to see if the underlying symptoms have improved. When tapering medication, it is important to distinguish recurrence of the original symptoms from transient rebound or withdrawal symptoms.

An alternative to benzodiazepines for GAD is buspirone. Buspirone is typically started at 5 mg tid. Average effective dosages are 30 mg/day in 3 divided doses, although total doses of up to 60 mg/day have been used. Buspirone is a good initial choice in detoxified alcoholic patients who may be at increased risk for benzodiazepine abuse.

Panic Attacks and Panic Disorder

The core manifestation of panic disorder is recurrent unexpected panic attacks. In addition, a substantial proportion of patients with panic disorder develop anticipatory anxiety and phobic avoidance, which may prove more disabling than the panic attacks themselves. When severe, phobic avoidance in the form of agoraphobia (fear of situations in which it may be difficult to gain help or escape) may cause patients to become entirely housebound.

Optimal therapy involves prevention of panic attacks and treatment of residual anticipatory anxiety and phobic avoidance symptoms. The most effective treatments for the prevention of panic attacks are pharmacologic and include the selective serotonin reuptake inhibitors (SSRIs), tricyclic antidepressants including clomipramine, MAOIs (see Chap. 3), and the high-potency benzodiazepines. Benzodiazepines may also be useful in the treatment of anticipatory anxiety and phobic avoidance, although nonpharmacologic treatments, especially behavior therapy, appear to be the treatments of choice. Patients with severe agoraphobia may be unable to leave their homes to attend treatment without short-term benzodiazepine therapy.

If they could be given in adequate doses, it is possible that all benzodiazepines might prove effective in preventing panic attacks; however, the required doses of lower-potency compounds, such as diazepam, would be so high as to produce marked oversedation. Therefore, only the high-potency compounds are clinically useful for this indication. The high-potency benzodiazepines that have been most clearly established as effective for panic disorder are the short-acting compound alprazolam and the long-acting compound clonazepam. There is some evidence to support the clinical utility of lorazepam as well.

Alprazolam is generally administered in dosages of 2–6 mg/day, although dosages as high as 10 mg/day have been used. Because it has a short duration of action, it is usually given in 3–4 divided doses. A sustained-release preparation is being tested that would permit once a day dosing. Clonazepam is generally used in dosages of 1–4 mg/day usually divided into 2 daily doses, although total daily doses as low as 0.5 and as high as 6.0 mg/day have been used. Clonazepam has some advantages and disadvantages with respect to alprazolam. The major problem with alprazolam is twofold: (1) It has a tendency to produce dependence with significant rebound and withdrawal symptoms. Thus, it may be very difficult to stop treatment with alprazolam after a therapeutic trial or successful course of treatment. (2) Because of its short half-life, a substantial minority of patients develop interdose rebound anxiety. Despite frequent doses throughout the day, such patients may endure a great deal of distress as the effects of the last dose wear off, leading to clock watching and, potentially, dosage acceleration. The availability of a sustained-release form of alprazolam may address the latter difficulty.

In some patients, it is easier to taper treatment with clonazepam than with alprazolam, perhaps because of its longer half-life, although the ultimate success of full discontinuation may not differ between the two drugs. The long half-life of clonazepam makes interdose rebound uncommon. Patients unable to wean themselves from alprazolam or patients with severe interdose rebound anxiety on alprazolam might do well to switch to clonazepam (method described on p. 175). A possible disadvantage of clonazepam is that it may be more commonly associated with the emergence of depression than alprazolam. This observation remains anecdotal, and the emergence of depression has also been reported during treatment with alprazolam.

The availability of multiple drug therapies for panic disorder permits the clinician to tailor treatment individually. An antidepressant might be chosen for a patient with a history of drug or alcohol abuse or of recurrent depression. A benzodiazepine might be chosen for patients extremely intolerant of medication side effects or when a more rapid clinical response is needed. In many situations, however, the clinician will have a wide range of choices. The advantage of benzodiazepines is the ease of starting therapy (i.e., rapid effect and few side effects beyond temporary sedation). The disadvantages become clearer later in therapy, when many patients find it difficult to discontinue benzodiazepines. The optimal duration of therapy for panic disorder with benzodiazepines or antidepressants is unknown, but it makes sense to try to taper pharmacologic therapy after 6 months of being symptom-free. Many patients with panic disorder, however, have a history of vulnerability to anxiety symptoms across the life cycle, beginning with inhibited behavior in early childhood, separation anxiety and school avoidance, social anxiety in adolescence, and panic attacks in early adulthood; these individuals also have family histories of anxiety disorders and more comorbidity with anxiety disorders. It is unrealistic to expect these patients to continue to feel and function as well over time without treatment in contrast to those with a more defined, acute syndrome, which more often remits with treatment.

Simple Phobias

Benzodiazepines are generally not the treatment of choice for simple phobias (fear of particular things, like spiders, airplanes, or heights). Behavior therapies appear to be successful with few contraindications. Nonetheless, if a patient with a phobia must confront the phobic stimulus on a particular occasion (e.g., an airplane flight), one-time use of a benzodiazepine (1–2 mg of lorazepam or 5–10 mg of diazepam) may be helpful.

Obsessive-Compulsive Disorder

Benzodiazepines are not generally effective in obsessive-compulsive disorder, although case series and one clinical trial indicated efficacy of clonazepam compared to placebo. This disorder is best treated with clomipramine or high doses of an SSRI in combination with behavior therapy (see Chap. 3). Clonazepam has been used adjunctively with these agents for incomplete responders. Buspirone was initially reported to be an effective adjunct to fluoxetine in the treatment of obsessive-compulsive disorder, but this result has not stood up in a subsequent well-designed study.

Depression

Benzodiazepines are not effective as primary treatments for major depressive illness, even when anxiety is a prominent symptom. Alprazolam has been reported to be as effective an antidepressant as imipramine in some patients; however, there have also been studies that found alprazolam to be less effective than cyclic antidepressants. In some studies that found alprazolam to be as effective as tricyclic antidepressants, the dosage of the tricyclic was too low, or the follow-up period was not long enough to see emergent differences between imipramine and alprazolam reach statistical significance. In clinical practice, alprazolam is not as effective as SSRIs, bupropion, venlafaxine, tricyclic antidepressants, or MAOIs. In addition, it carries the risk of dependence, which the antidepressants do not. Alprazolam should not be considered a primary treatment for depression.

Depression with Anxiety

When anxiety is a prominent symptom of depressive illness, temporary adjunctive use of a benzodiazepine (1–4 weeks) may be helpful while waiting for the onset of action of the antidepressant. It should be emphasized that benzodiazepines are not a substitute for effective antidepressant treatment and that patients should be instructed about the short-term nature of benzodiazepine therapy (see Chap. 3).

Depression with Insomnia

Patients with major depressive illness often have trouble sleeping. However, many of the antidepressants with the most favorable side effect profiles (e.g., the SSRIs, venlafaxine, desipramine, nortriptyline, and bupropion) are nonsedating or may even cause insomnia as a side effect (e.g., SSRIs, bupropion, or tranylcypromine). The clinician may approach depression with insomnia in one of two ways—either by relying on a more sedating antidepressant compound, such as imipramine or doxepin (with the entire dose given at bedtime), at the expense of anticholinergic and possible cardiovascular side effects, or with temporary use of a sedative-hypnotic at bedtime in addition to the antidepressant. Benzodiazepines and trazodone (50 mg hs; see Chap. 3) are the most widely used sedatives for this purpose. As with any clinical situation in which drugs are used for symptomatic relief of certain aspects of an illness (e.g., aspirin for fever), benzodiazepines should not be allowed to interfere with primary treatment. In general, the duration of their use should be limited (e.g., 1–3 weeks) pending the therapeutic response to the antidepressant. Longer-term use of a benzodiazepine or adjunctive trazodone will only be necessary when the patient is having a good response to the primary antidepressant (e.g., fluoxetine) but is having continued serious insomnia as a side effect of that antidepressant.

Insomnia

Insomnia is a common symptom that can result from a wide variety of causes. Insomnia should be thoroughly investigated prior to prescribing a benzodiazepine for symptomatic treatment. It is important to determine the onset, duration, and nature of the sleep disturbance, to review the medical and psychiatric histories, with special attention to medication, caffeine, alcohol, or other drug use, and to perform a physical and mental status examination. While insomnia often proves to be idiopathic or due to an identifiable transient stress, difficulty in sleeping is not infrequently a symptom of serious medical or psychiatric disorder, such as depression or alcoholism, or of a specific sleep disorder (Table 6-5). Clinically, insomnia of only a few days' duration is most often the result of pain, situational anxiety, stress, or drug or medication use. Insomnia lasting more than 3 weeks is more likely to be secondary to a medical or psychiatric disorder.

For short-term insomnia, benzodiazepines are effective symptomatic treatments, but should follow the use of nonpharmacologic interventions: (1) Patients should be advised to stop using alcohol or

Table 6-5.   Causes of insomnia

Common medically related
  Pain
  Respiratory problems such as chronic cough or paroxysmal nocturnal
    dyspnea
  Nocturnal angina
  Hyperthyroidism
  Esophageal reflux, diarrhea, and other gastrointestinal complaints
  Nocturia
Drug and alcohol related
  Chronic alcoholism
  Alcohol use prior to retiring
  Caffeine and other psychostimulant use
  Withdrawal from alcohol, sedative-hypnotics, or narcotics
  Discontinuation of hypnotic drugs
  Neuroleptic-induced akathisia
  SSRIs, bupropion tranylcypromine
Psychiatric disorder related
  Depression
  Mania
  Anxiety disorders (including posttraumatic stress disorder)
  Dementing disorders, especially with superimposed delirium
Specific sleep disorder related
  Sleep apnea (obstructive or central)
  Nocturnal myoclonus
  Restless legs syndrome
Environmental and behavioral related
  Change in sleeping environment
  Current life stress
  Preoccupation with falling asleep
  Air travel across time zones
Idiopathic

stimulants such as caffeine near bedtime; (2) excessive and inappropriate medications should be withdrawn; (3) patients should be instructed not to nap during the day; (4) the patient's bedroom should be sufficiently dark and quiet; (5) important life stressors should be ascertained and addressed; and (6) any obsessional overconcern with sleep that might contribute to insomnia must be addressed.

If prescribing a benzodiazepine, a small amount should be given, usually no more than a 2-week supply. For long-term insomnia for which no primary medical or psychiatric cause can be found, long-term use of benzodiazepines may also be helpful, but the ratio of benefit (long-term efficacy) to risk (dependence, impairment of psychomotor performance, subtle changes in mood) has not been clearly established.

The greatest benefit of benzodiazepines appears to be reduced sleep fragmentation during the night. In addition, benzodiazepines have many effects of unknown clinical significance: They suppress REM sleep, prolong REM latency, increase stage 2 sleep, and decrease stages 1, 3, and 4 sleep. Flurazepam, temazepam, triazolam, quazepam, estazolam, and the nonbenzodiazepine zolpidem are specifically marketed for insomnia, although, as noted, the benzodiazepine hypnotics have no special features to distinguish them from other benzodiazepines such as diazepam. Outside the United States, a variety of other benzodiazepines are marketed as hypnotics, including brotizolam, loprazolam, lormetazepam, and nitrazepam. The nonbenzodiazepine zolpidem has little effect on stages of sleep perhaps because of its binding profile for a subset of benzodiazepine receptors. Whether this offers unique clinical benefits is unknown but is potentially an advantage.

In healthy adults, the standard hypnotic dose of flurazepam and temazepam is 30 mg, although 15 mg is effective for some individuals. Quazepam is given at 15 mg; 7.5 mg may be adequate for some individuals and is the manufacturer's recommended dose for the elderly. Because of the risk of accumulation, flurazepam and quazepam should not be used in the elderly if more than a few days' use is contemplated, in which case temazepam, 15 mg, would be a better choice. Triazolam is given at 0.125–0.25 mg nightly (0.125 mg in the elderly). Zolpidem is available as a 10-mg tablet for usual adult dosing, but the 5-mg strength should be selected for the elderly.

The two major concerns in choosing a benzodiazepine hypnotic are rapidity of onset and half-life. For patients who report difficulty in falling asleep, the rapidity of onset of the drug is particularly important. After oral administration, diazepam and flurazepam act rapidly, achieving peak plasma concentrations in 0.5–1.0 hour. Triazolam (1.3 hours to peak) and quazepam (1.5 hours to peak) have intermediate rates of absorption. Temazepam has a slower rate of onset, with peak levels achieved after only 3 hours, making it less helpful for sleep-latency insomnia unless taken 1 hour prior to bedtime. To improve absorption, all benzodiazepines should be administered on an empty stomach.

The other important consideration in choosing a hypnotic is half-life. Flurazepam has a long-lived metabolite, N-desalkylflurazepam (see Fig. 6-3), which reaches its peak plasma concentration approximately 10 hours after an oral dose. After 2 weeks of nightly administration, this metabolite (which has a half-life of 50–160 hours [200 hours or more in the elderly]) accumulates to levels 7–8 times its peak level on the first night. Although only 3.5% of N-desalkylflurazepam is free (not protein-bound), after 2 weeks this represents a great deal of pharmacodynamic activity; indeed, with repeat dosing, this metabolite may represent most of the active compound in plasma. Quazepam is metabolized to oxoquazepam and then to N-desalkylflurazepam, which, as in the case of flurazepam, represents most of the drug's pharmacodynamic activity with chronic dosing. With repetitive administration, this drug is not likely to differ significantly from flurazepam in its effects. However, at the time of this writing, it was significantly more expensive.

Two advantages of long-acting drugs are that they may decrease early morning awakening and treat daytime anxiety. However, the trade-off may be residual daytime drowsiness, possible neuropsychiatric impairment, and possible interactions with other CNS depressants, such as ethanol, that might be consumed during the day (although most patients develop tolerance to daytime effects and experience no "hangover" and little impairment). In the elderly, the level of accumulation may be such as to produce intoxication or delirium; therefore, in the elderly, repetitive dosing with long-acting compounds, such as flurazepam, quazepam, or diazepam, is not recommended.

Short-acting drugs do not accumulate but may cause rebound insomnia. Rebound insomnia may occur when short-acting benzodiazepines (e.g., triazolam, alprazolam, or lorazepam) are used on several consecutive nights. The shortest period necessary to produce rebound is unclear, but it may be only several days. Rebound is common when triazolam is used at dosages of 0.5 mg nightly; it is less of a problem at a dosage of 0.25 mg nightly but is still reported by many patients. On the first or second night after discontinuation of short-acting benzodiazepines, patients may complain of increased sleep latency and increased total wake time. After discontinuing triazolam, 0.5 mg, there may be a 25% reduction in total sleep time on the first night after discontinuation. Especially if misinterpreted as reemergence of underlying chronic insomnia, rebound may reinforce chronic benzodiazepine use and risk of dependence. In addition to rebound after discontinuation, triazolam, which has a very short half-life, may cause rebound symptoms within the same night, manifested by early morning awakening and morning anxiety symptoms. Rebound side effects from triazolam may occur even if it was ineffective for the original complaint of insomnia. Rebound insomnia appears to be uncommon with temazepam and with very long-acting drugs such as flurazepam. If rebound insomnia occurs with flurazepam, it might not be expected until 4–10 nights after discontinuation. Because of its short half-life, rebound is to be expected with zolpidem.

Barbiturates, such as secobarbital, pentobarbital, and amobarbital, and related drugs, glutethimide and ethchlorvynol, essentially have no place in the treatment of insomnia because of their high risk of causing tolerance and dependence and their danger in overdose. Of the barbiturate-like drugs, chloral hydrate appears to be the least problematic, with relatively low abuse potential. Thus, it is still used as an alternative to benzodiazepines by some physicians. For patients with a history of adverse reactions to benzodiazepines or a history of alcohol or sedative-hypnotic abuse, sedating antihistamines are sometimes used, but they are less effective in reducing sleep latency than benzodiazepines and are associated with residual daytime sedation and anticholinergic effects. Diphenhydramine is most commonly used, often at a dose of 50 mg (range 25–100 mg). Its half-life is 3.4–9.3 hours. Hydroxyzine, with a half-life of 7–20 hours, and doxylamine, with a half-life of 4–12 hours, are also sometimes used as hypnotics. All sedating antihistamines are strongly anticholinergic and should not be prescribed in combination with other anticholinergic compounds. It is important to monitor elderly patients for emergence of anticholinergic toxicity. The sedating antidepressants amitriptyline, doxepin, and trazodone have often been used in low dosages (e.g., 25–50 mg nightly) for primary insomnia. They have not been well studied for primary insomnia with respect to efficacy and the development of tachyphylaxis, but they may be safe in sleep apnea (although this is not fully established). The disadvantages, at least of the tricyclics amitriptyline and doxepin, are that they are strongly anticholinergic, are dangerous in overdose, and have cardiac side effects (see Chap. 3). Trazodone-50 has been shown to be better than placebo in treatment of insomnia induced by SSRIs or bupropion.

Alcohol Withdrawal

Because of their effectiveness and safety, benzodiazepines are the agents of choice for the treatment of withdrawal from ethanol. The effectiveness of benzodiazepines is based on their pharmacologic cross-tolerance with ethanol.

Mechanism of Action

Benzodiazepines and ethanol increase activation of $GABA_A$ receptors. With chronic high-dose ethanol (or barbiturate or benzodiazepine) use, there is an apparent decrease in efficacy of $GABA_A$ receptors (a mechanism of tolerance and dependence). When high-dose ethanol is discontinued, this "down-regulated" state of GABAergic transmission is unmasked. Gamma-aminobutyric acid is the most important inhibitory neurotransmitter in the brain; therefore, this state is manifested by anxiety, insomnia, agitated delirium, and a tendency to have seizures. By augmenting the effectiveness of GABA at its $GABA_A$ receptors, benzodiazepines restore adequate CNS inhibition. Slow withdrawal of the benzodiazepine detoxification agent presumably permits recovery of GABAergic systems to normal levels of activity.

Clinical Indications

Benzodiazepine treatment of alcohol withdrawal helps with anxiety, agitation, insomnia, and autonomic symptoms, and it may prevent seizures. Additionally benzodiazepines make patients more comfortable and therefore more likely to complete detoxification. Adequate benzodiazepine therapy may also prevent progression to the life-threatening syndrome delirium tremens. Benzodiazepines are therefore especially important for patients at high risk for delirium tremens, including those with a complicating medical illness, malnutrition, dehydration, or a prior history of delirium tremens. Should delirium emerge, benzodiazepines are effective sedatives.

Once a diagnosis of alcohol withdrawal has been established, aggressive treatment is indicated for hypertension, tachycardia, tremulousness, agitation, and other objective signs of withdrawal. Ideally, a calm state should be produced as swiftly as possible without making the patient excessively drowsy. All benzodiazepines are probably effective in the treatment of alcohol withdrawal, provided that an adequate dosage is used. Patients with hepatic dysfunction should be treated with either oxazepam or lorazepam; these short-acting benzodiazepines are metabolized by glucuronidation (a metabolic pathway that is relatively preserved in liver disease), and they have no active metabolites. Other patients are probably best served by using a long-acting benzodiazepine, such as chlordiazepoxide or diazepam, because these drugs minimize the chance that symptoms will emerge between doses and because long-acting drugs are usually easier to taper than short-acting ones.

Dosing

Whenever possible, benzodiazepine dosages should be adjusted to control symptoms rather than keeping to an arbitrary dosage schedule because the dosages required to achieve adequate sedation vary markedly. For example, some patients may require 2000 mg of chlordiazepoxide on the first day, whereas others may be oversedated by a dose of 200 mg. Oral doses in the range of 25–100 mg of chlordiazepoxide or 5–20 mg of diazepam, q4h prn, are usually effective in the treatment of withdrawal symptoms.

Other Drugs for Withdrawal

The beta-adrenergic blocker atenolol has been reported to be an effective adjunct to benzodiazepines in the treatment of alcohol withdrawal (see Chap. 7). Since it does not produce cross-tolerance with alcohol, beta-adrenergic blockers cannot replace benzodiazepines as sole agents of detoxification. Preliminary studies also suggest a possible role for carbamazepine in alcohol withdrawal (see Chap. 5). Antipsychotic drugs cannot substitute for benzodiazepines. High-potency antipsychotic drugs (e.g., haloperidol, 5 mg) may be useful in the emergency treatment of intoxicated belligerent alcoholics. High-potency antipsychotics may also be useful in the treatment of alcoholic hallucinosis (i.e., auditory, visual, or tactile hallucinations caused by alcohol withdrawal); however, benzodiazepines will still be required for the remainder of the withdrawal symptomatology. Low-potency antipsychotic drugs, such as chlorpromazine and thioridazine, should be avoided during alcohol withdrawal because of their adverse effect on the seizure threshold and their tendency to precipitate postural hypotension.

Delirium Tremens

Once a patient develops "full-blown" delirium tremens, with hypertension, fever, and delirium, symptoms may be very difficult to control. The development of this syndrome constitutes a medical emergency, as it carries a substantial risk of mortality. Preferably, patients should be treated in an intensive care setting. In addition to supportive care and workup for other medical illnesses (e.g., pneumonia or subdural hematoma), aggressive use of benzodiazepines is indicated. Benzodiazepines should be given IV if possible to ensure absorption. Lorazepam, 2 mg q2h, or diazepam, 5–10 mg q2h, can be used as starting dosages. The final dosages used should be a function of the patient's symptoms and not based on any arbitrary maximum dosage. Risk of oversedation is greatest if repeated dosing is given before the prior dosage has reached peak effect.

Use in Mania and Psychotic Disorders

Acute Mania and Other Agitated Psychoses

Several small studies and case reports have suggested that clonazepam may be effective for acute mania either as a sole agent or in combination with lithium; there have also been negative reports. To date there is no convincing evidence that clonazepam has a specific antimanic action. Clonazepam and other benzodiazepines do have a role as adjunctive sedatives in the treatment of mania, as described below.

Many patients with mania and other psychoses require sedation, especially early in the course of illness. Benzodiazepines are safe and reliable sedatives that are relatively free of side effects. Benzodiazepines should not be permitted to interfere with the primary treatment, which will consist of a mood stabilizer or an antipsychotic drug depending on the diagnosis. However, benzodiazepines have advantages over prn use of antipsychotic drugs for acute control of dangerous or hyperactive behavior (see also Acute Psychosis, p. 24). Although prn doses of antipsychotic drugs have frequently been used for control of disruptive behavior and hyperactivity, these drugs have many side effects, including akathisia, which may worsen the patient's agitation. A sample regimen using benzodiazepines might be haloperidol, 5 mg bid, with lorazepam, 1–2 mg PO or IM q2h prn, or clonazepam, 0.5–1.0 mg PO q2h prn, until a calming effect is achieved. The interval between doses can then be extended. Benzodiazepines can generally be tapered within 2–3 weeks, thus making dependence unlikely.

Bipolar Prophylaxis

For bipolar prophylaxis, in one retrospective study of patients requiring both lithium and antipsychotics (Sachs et al., 1990), clonazepam, 0.5–3.0 mg/day, successfully replaced the antipsychotic drugs in 6 of 17 bipolar patients (lithium therapy was continued unchanged). A less satisfactory outcome was found in a prospective study (Aronson et al., 1989) in which antipsychotics were replaced by clonazepam, 2–5 mg/day, while lithium was continued. The trial was terminated after only five patients were enrolled because all patients relapsed rapidly, one within 2 weeks and four within 10–15 weeks.

At present, the utility of clonazepam for bipolar prophylaxis is unclear, but for patients who cannot be managed with mood stabilizers alone it is worth trying to replace antipsychotic medication with clonazepam. Even if this works only in a minority of patients, it could prove to be a useful intervention by decreasing the risk of tardive dyskinesia. Like other benzodiazepines, clonazepam has been associated with the emergence of depression in patients being treated for a variety of disorders. Whether this represents a toxic effect or simply an inability to prevent depression is unknown.

Catatonic Symptoms

Parenteral lorazepam has been reported to reverse both neuroleptic-induced and psychogenic catatonia. Doses of 1–2 mg IV or 2 mg IM have been reported to produce rapid and dramatic reversal of catatonic states. Although the percentage of catatonic patients who actually respond to lorazepam is unknown, it is reasonable to try lorazepam in catatonia because it is relatively safe when given IM or slowly IV (safer than amobarbital). This may be an especially useful option for patients in whom it is unclear whether the catatonic syndrome is the result of neuroleptics and from whom neuroleptics should therefore be withheld. Because lorazepam has multiple effects on the nervous system, its effectiveness does not clarify the diagnosis. For example, lorazepam might also be effective if apparent catatonia was due to complex partial status epilepticus.

Long-Term Use in Chronic Nonaffective Psychoses

Benzodiazepines are commonly administered as long-term adjuncts to antipsychotic drugs during the chronic phase of schizophrenia and other psychotic disorders. Although this indication has not been well studied in a controlled fashion, it appears from case reports and clinical practice that judicious use of benzodiazepines may improve anxiety related to the psychotic disorder and may also decrease neuroleptic-induced akathisia. Although some clinicians have found the high-potency compound alprazolam partially effective for ameliorating negative (deficit) symptoms of schizophrenia, use of long-acting low-potency benzodiazepines, such as diazepam, may be advantageous because of their lower risk of producing dependence.

Symptomatic Treatment of Agitated Delirium

The key to treating delirium is supportive care while specific therapy for the underlying disorder is given. However, symptomatic treatment with sedatives is often necessary when no cause for the delirium can be found or while awaiting the effect of specific therapy. Because delirious patients are unpredictable, restraints are generally indicated. When used, sedatives should be given at the lowest effective dosage. Delirium due to ethanol withdrawal is best managed with a benzodiazepine. Delirium due to withdrawal from barbiturate-like drugs is best managed with phenobarbital, although long-acting benzodiazepines may also be used. In other types of delirium, especially in the elderly, the high-potency antipsychotic drug haloperidol may be preferable because it is less likely than benzodiazepines to produce inattention, thereby worsening confusion. Haloperidol also has little effect on cardiorespiratory status (see Chap. 2).

If haloperidol is ineffective or not tolerated, a benzodiazepine could be used; lorazepam and oxazepam are good choices because they have short half-lives, have no active metabolites, and are metabolized by glucuronidation, which is relatively preserved in the elderly and in cirrhosis. Lorazepam has the advantage of a parenteral form and more rapid absorption when given orally. Lorazepam can be given intramuscularly with reliable absorption or intravenously. The very short-acting benzodiazepine midazolam is also sometimes used for sedation, but if repeat administration is contemplated, a longer-acting compound would be preferable.

Depending on the patient's age and degree of agitation, lorazepam, 0.5–2.0 mg, can be given slowly IV; slow administration avoids the production of high peak levels that could cause respiratory arrest. Nonetheless, intravenous benzodiazepines should only be given if personnel trained in cardiopulmonary resuscitation are present. The dose of lorazepam can be repeated q20min until the patient is sedated. Repeat dosing thereafter should be on a prn basis q2h. Combinations of haloperidol and lorazepam may be quite useful in patients with marked hallucinations and delusions who remain hyperactive after large doses of haloperidol or who develop extrapyramidal symptoms on higher doses of haloperidol. In these patients, it is best to administer a fixed dose of haloperidol daily and then to titrate the level of sedation.

Neuroleptic-Induced Akathisia

Akathisia is an uncomfortable side effect of neuroleptics described by patients as a subjective need to be in motion and characterized behaviorally by motor restlessness. Akathisia may produce severe agitation and lead to treatment refusal. (Treatment of akathisia is fully discussed in Chap. 2.) When a benzodiazepine is used, diazepam, 5 mg tid, or lorazepam, 1 mg tid, may be effective. When an effective dose is found, a response is seen within 1–2 days.

METHOD OF USE

Starting Therapy

Prior to starting a benzodiazepine, patients should be cautioned about possible sedation and warned not to drive vehicles or operate dangerous machinery until it is determined that their dose does not affect performance. Patients should be instructed to take their medication on an empty stomach and not concomitantly with antacids because meals and antacids may decrease absorption. No specific laboratory tests are required before beginning benzodiazepines. A prior history of alcohol or other substance abuse is a relative contraindication to the use of benzodiazepines; a compelling indication, lack of an effective alternative, and careful supervision are required in this population. An alternative for the detoxified alcoholic with GAD is buspirone or an antidepressant. Active alcoholics should not be treated for a putative anxiety disorder until they are detoxified.

For short-term treatment of situational anxiety, total doses of more than 30 mg of diazepam or the equivalent are almost never needed. Higher doses are occasionally needed in generalized anxiety disorder. For sleep, 30 mg of flurazepam, 30 mg of temazepam, 5 mg of diazepam, 15 mg of quazepam, 1 mg of lorazepam, or 0.25 mg of triazolam is the average starting dose for healthy adults. In the elderly, lower doses and avoidance of long-acting drugs should be the rule.

When benzodiazepines are used as anxiolytics, low doses (e.g., diazepam, 5 mg tid) should be used initially to avoid oversedation. The dosage can be slowly increased until a therapeutic effect occurs. Dosage changes with long-acting drugs (e.g., diazepam, chlordiazepoxide, or clorazepate) should be slow because the drugs reach steady state levels over a period of a week or more. Dosages of short-acting drugs (e.g., lorazepam or oxazepam) can be increased more rapidly (e.g., after two days).

In follow-up, patients should be asked not only about effectiveness but also about side effects. Patients who complain of sedation may do better with a temporary dosage reduction; there is some evidence that, over time, many individuals develop tolerance to sedative effects. Since the plasma levels of benzodiazepines that result in sedation are only about twice as high as those levels that are anxiolytic, some patients being treated for anxiety may do better on multiple low doses during the day rather than fewer and larger doses. Frequent (tid–qid) lower doses result in less fluctuation in plasma levels than occurs with less frequent dosing, in which the patient might experience oversedation at peak levels and inadequate treatment at troughs. Patients on short-acting compounds such as alprazolam should be questioned about interdose rebound anxiety.

If a given benzodiazepine produces intolerable side effects or fails to be helpful after 2–3 weeks, the difficulty may derive from the pharmacokinetic profile, and if so, another benzodiazepine can be tried, preferably one with a different pharmacokinetic profile. Alternatively, another class of drugs may be tried (e.g., buspirone or an antidepressant for GAD or an antidepressant for panic disorder).

Tolerance and Discontinuation Symptoms

The benzodiazepines may induce dependence, with a risk of producing clinically significant symptomatology on discontinuation. Discontinuation symptoms can be conceptually divided into (1) recurrence of the original disorder, (2) rebound (a marked temporary return of original symptoms), and (3) withdrawal (recurrence of the original symptoms plus new symptoms such as tachycardia or hypertension). In clinical practice, these syndromes demonstrate a great deal of overlap and frequently coexist. The nature of the symptoms and their time course may help in making distinctions.

Recurrences generally emerge slowly and do not subside with time; the symptoms are generally indistinguishable from those present prior to treatment. Recurrences are frequent in panic disorder. Generally, the response to recurrence of the original disorder is resumption of therapy.

Rebound symptoms occur soon after discontinuation and generally represent a temporary return of original symptoms, such as anxiety or insomnia, but at a greater intensity than the original symptoms. The response to rebound symptoms is to wait them out if they are mild or to resume therapy and then taper the benzodiazepine more slowly. For some high-potency compounds with a short half-life, such as alprazolam and triazolam, rebound symptoms may occur even during maintenance therapy as blood levels between doses reach their nadir. If interdose rebound symptoms or rebound occurring with attempts to decrease the dosage represents a serious clinical problem, a switch to a compound with a longer half-life may prove helpful.

The onset of **withdrawal** symptoms generally reflects the half-life of the drug used—usually 1–2 days for short-acting drugs, 2–5 days for long-acting drugs (although symptoms beginning as late as 7–10 days have been reported). Withdrawal symptoms generally peak several days after onset and slowly disappear over 1–3 weeks. In contrast to recurrence and rebound, withdrawal syndromes include symptoms that the patient has not previously experienced. Benzodiazepine withdrawal symptoms include anxiety, irritability, insomnia, tremulousness, sweating, anorexia, nausea, diarrhea, abdominal discomfort, lethargy, fatigue, tachycardia, systolic hypertension, delirium, and seizures.

The risk of developing dependence and thus rebound and withdrawal symptoms is higher with long-term treatment, higher doses, and higher-potency drugs. The likelihood and severity of rebound and withdrawal symptoms also reflect the half-life of the compound; such symptoms occur more frequently and are generally more severe with compounds with a short half-life. In thinking about the risks of dependence and discontinuation syndromes, the benzodiazepines can be subdivided into four groups, those with

1. High potency and short duration of action: alprazolam, estazolam, midazolam, lorazepam, and triazolam
2. High potency and long duration of action: clonazepam
3. Low potency and short duration of action: oxazepam and temazepam
4. Low potency and long duration of action: chlordiazepoxide, clorazepate, diazepam, flurazepam, halazepam, and quazepam

No withdrawal syndrome has been detected for buspirone.

Although dependence can be induced by any benzodiazepine, with low-potency, long-acting drugs, dependence is relatively uncommon in the therapeutic setting (although dependence readily occurs with very high doses). In addition, with this group of compounds, rebound and withdrawal symptoms are typically mild and self-limited when they occur. Dependence is most likely and rebound and withdrawal symptoms are most severe with high-potency, short-acting benzodiazepines, such as alprazolam, lorazepam, and triazolam. These are the compounds that are most likely to produce delirium and seizures after abrupt discontinuation from high doses. In addition to the more common benzodiazepine withdrawal symptoms, severe dysphoria and psychotic-like symptoms have been reported in patients discontinuing alprazolam. Because they are atypical, these symptoms may be extremely confusing on presentation unless a history of alprazolam discontinuation is obtained.

For some patients, discontinuation of alprazolam may be easier via a switch to equipotent doses of a longer-acting high-potency benzodiazepine such as clonazepam (see next section). A small number of reports have also suggested that carbamazepine may be a useful adjunct for alprazolam withdrawal. While this strategy may aid an individual patient, a large controlled study failed to show evidence of efficacy.

Many sedative drugs share cross-tolerance with the benzodiazepines, including barbiturates, meprobamate, alcohols, propanediols, aldehydes, glutethimide, methyprylon, and methaqualone. Buspirone does not produce cross-tolerance with benzodiazepines, ethanol, or barbiturates and is not useful in withdrawal from these drugs.

Problems with benzodiazepine tolerance, rebound, and withdrawal can be minimized if low-potency, long-acting compounds are used whenever possible (e.g., in the treatment of generalized anxiety disorder). If long-acting compounds are relatively contraindicated (e.g., in the elderly or in patients who develop excessive sedation with repeated dosing), use of low-potency, short-acting compounds may represent an alternative (e.g., temazepam for the treatment of insomnia). However, it must be recalled that at high doses, even low-potency compounds may cause serious discontinuation symptomatology. As with any drug that is being discontinued after a protracted period of use, gradual tapering of benzodiazepines is the most judicious approach. Probably the greatest dangers from benzodiazepine withdrawal occur when patients on short-acting drugs stop their medication suddenly without consulting their physician.

Switching from Alprazolam to Clonazepam

Despite the clear efficacy of alprazolam for panic disorder, there are clinical circumstances in which it is indicated to switch patients from alprazolam to another high-potency benzodiazepine. These circumstances include serious interdose rebound anxiety (symptom recurrence after an increasingly short period and early morning anxiety prior to the first daily dose) and difficulty with tapering and discontinuing alprazolam. As described previously, both of these circumstances reflect the high potency and short half-life of alprazolam. Switching to clonazepam appears to address these clinical problems because clonazepam is potent enough to replace alprazolam but has a long half-life (2–4 days). A method of switching was reported by Herman and associates (1987) based on a study of 48 patients with panic disorder. The switch takes approximately 1 week (the minimum time to reach a steady state level of clonazepam). A sustained-release formulation of alprazolam may minimize these concerns and offer an alternative to switching to clonazepam.

1. Clonazepam is given at one-half the total daily alprazolam dose divided into an early morning and a mid-afternoon dose.
2. Regular alprazolam doses are stopped, but during the first 7 days, alprazolam can be taken as needed up to the full amount taken previously.

3. Alprazolam is stopped entirely after day 7.
4. If more medication is needed after day 7, clonazepam is increased by 0.25–0.5 mg every week until efficacy is reestablished.

Abuse

Contrary to public impressions, it appears that very few patients who have received benzodiazepines for valid indications become abusers (i.e., increase their dosage without medical supervision and take the drugs for nonmedical purposes). Most abusers of benzodiazepines also abuse other drugs. Serious abusers of CNS depressants may use the equivalent of hundreds of milligrams of diazepam per day. Serious CNS depressant abusers should be detoxified as inpatients using either phenobarbital or a long-acting benzodiazepine, such as diazepam, as the detoxification agent.

USE IN THE ELDERLY

Slowed hepatic metabolism and increased pharmacodynamic sensitivity mean that great care must be taken when prescribing benzodiazepines in the elderly. In general, short-acting benzodiazepines are safest, especially those metabolized by glucuronidation alone (lorazepam, temazepam, and oxazepam). In one study of patients over age 65, use of benzodiazepines with an elimination half-life of more than 24 hours, but not benzodiazepines with a short half-life, was associated with a 70% increase in the risk of hip fracture compared with individuals not using any psychotropic drugs (Ray et al., 1989). Although the results of this study did not achieve statistical significance and require replication, they deserve attention because the risk of hip fracture also increased with higher doses, suggesting that the observed effect was real. Accumulation of long-acting benzodiazepines must always be considered in the differential diagnosis of delirium or rapid cognitive decline in the elderly.

USE IN PREGNANCY

Earlier reports associating diazepam with both cleft lip and cleft palate have not been substantiated. On the other hand, there are no prospective studies to demonstrate that benzodiazepines are safe during pregnancy. One recent report described intra- and extrauterine growth restriction, dysmorphism, and CNS dysfunction as a result of intrauterine benzodiazepine exposure, but the study was compromised by biased patient selection and failure to control adequately for use of other psychotropic drugs. Although there is no convincing evidence that benzodiazepines are teratogenic, it would be wise to avoid benzodiazepines, especially early in pregnancy (oral cleft closure is usually complete by the tenth gestational week), unless there are compelling indications for their use.

SIDE EFFECTS AND TOXICITY

The benzodiazepines have little effect on autonomic function, unlike certain antipsychotic and antidepressant drugs. Thus, adverse effects on blood pressure, pulse, and cardiac rhythm are not typically seen. Benzodiazepines may produce slow-wave and low-voltage fast (beta) activity on electroencephalographic testing that is without clinical consequence.

Sedation and Impairment of Performance
Fatigue and drowsiness are the most common side effects associated with benzodiazepine treatment. In addition, impairment of memory and recall, reduced motor coordination, and impairment of cognitive function may occur. The development of these side effects depends on dosage employed, concomitant use of other medications, especially CNS depressants, and alcohol, and the sensitivity of the individual being treated. With repeated dosing, as would occur with the treatment of anxiety disorders, most patients develop tolerance to sedation. The suggestion that automobile accidents are more likely to occur among benzodiazepine users is complicated by the possibility that the condition being treated (e.g., anxiety, insomnia) may be a contributing factor. The interpretation of laboratory studies of attention, intellectual function, reflexes, cognitive function, and driving ability is difficult to generalize to real life situations.

Effects on Memory
Acute dosages of benzodiazepines may produce transient anterograde amnesia. This effect appears to be independent of sedation; acquisition of new information is specifically impaired. The risk of anterograde amnesia appears to be worsened by concomitant ingestion of alcohol. Anterograde amnesia may be desirable when oral or parenteral benzodiazepines are given for preoperative sedation; however, anterograde amnesia is undesirable in most other circumstances. Short-acting, high-potency agents (e.g., triazolam) appear to be the worst offenders; there have been reports of serious amnesia in travelers who have used triazolam to sleep during flights across time zones. Given its potency and half-life, anterograde amnesia may occur with zolpidem as well. At present, there is inadequate experience to judge.

Disinhibition
Reports of paradoxical reactions to benzodiazepines (disinhibition) are not infrequent. Reports describing rage outbursts or aggression in patients on chlordiazepoxide, diazepam, alprazolam, or clonazepam have appeared. Increased impulsiveness, euphoria, and frank mania have been reported with alprazolam. Disinhibition can likely occur with any benzodiazepine, but there is suggestion that the lower-potency, slowly absorbed oxazepam may be less likely to trigger this effect. Many clinicians feel that the highest incidence of disinhibition occurs in personality disorder patients with prior histories of dyscontrol. When severely symptomatic dyscontrol occurs (e.g., in a patient who was given a benzodiazepine in an emergency room or inpatient ward), the administration of haloperidol, 5 mg IM, is often effective in producing sedation.

Depression
All benzodiazepines have been associated with the emergence or worsening of depression; whether they were causative or only failed to prevent the depression is unknown. While it makes sense to lower the dosage or discontinue the benzodiazepine when depression occurs during the course of benzodiazepine treatment, the addition of an antidepressant is typically very effective. If the depression occurs during the course of treatment for panic disorder, the benzodiazepine can be replaced by an antidepressant.

Table 6-6.   Interactions of benzodiazepines with other drugs

Decrease absorption
  Antacids
Increase central nervous system depression
  Antihistamines
  Barbiturates and similarly acting drugs
  Cyclic antidepressants
  Ethanol
Increase benzodiazepine levels (compete for microsomal enzymes; probably
    little or no effect on lorazepam, oxazepam, temazepam)
  Cimetidine
  Disulfiram
  Erythromycin
  Estrogens
  Isoniazid
  SSRIs
Decrease benzodiazepine levels
  Carbamazepine (possibly other anticonvulsants)

OVERDOSE

Benzodiazepines have proved to be remarkably safe in overdose. By themselves, only rarely have they been implicated in fatal overdoses, although when combined with other CNS depressants, such as alcohol, barbiturates, or narcotics, they may contribute to the lethality of the overdose. There have been some unsettling reports, however, of lethal overdoses with very high-potency benzodiazepines such as triazolam (e.g., Sunter et al., 1988). It is hard to interpret these reports, since alcohol or concurrent medical illness was involved in some cases. The replacement of barbiturates and related compounds by benzodiazepines has markedly decreased the number of successful suicides associated with sleeping pills.

The treatment of benzodiazepine overdose includes induction of emesis or gastric lavage, when appropriate, and supportive care for patients who are stuporous or comatose. The benzodiazepine antagonist flumazenil is available for the treatment of benzodiazepine overdose. In tolerant patients, this drug may precipitate withdrawal symptoms in analogy with the actions of naloxone in opiate-dependent individuals.

INTERACTIONS WITH ALCOHOL AND OTHER DRUGS

Serious pharmacokinetic drug interactions are rare with benzodiazepines but may occur (Table 6-6). Benzodiazepines can cause a mild to moderate increase in CNS depression caused by co-ingested alcohol; when taken together in overdose, ethanol and benzodiazepines can result in death.

BIBLIOGRAPHY

Pharmacokinetics

Greenblatt, D. J., Harmatz, J. S., Englehardt, N., and Shader, R. I. Pharmacokinetic determinants of dynamic differences among three benzodiazepine hypnotics. *Arch. Gen. Psychiatry* 46 : 326, 1989.
Greenblatt, D. J., Shader, R. I., and Koch-Weser, J. Slow absorption of intramuscular chlordiazepoxide. *N. Engl. J. Med.* 291 : 1116, 1974.

Salzman, C., Shader, R. I., Greenblatt, D. J., and Harmatz, J. S. Long vs. short half-life benzodiazepines in the elderly. *Arch. Gen. Psychiatry* 40 : 293, 1983.

Scavone, J. M., Greenblatt, D. J., and Shader, R. I. Alprazolam kinetics following sublingual and oral administration. *J. Clin. Psychopharmacol.* 7 : 332, 1987.

Mechanism of Action

Levitan, E. S., Schofield, P. R., Burt, D. R., et al. Structural and functional basis for GABA$_A$ receptor heterogeneity. *Nature* 335 : 76, 1988.

Pritchett, D. B., Sontheimer, H., Shivers, B., et al. Importance of a novel GABA$_A$ receptor subunit for benzodiazepine pharmacology. *Nature* 338 : 582, 1989.

Disorders Treated

Anxiety

Kahn, R. J., McNair, D. M., Lipman, R. S., et al. Imipramine and chlordiazepoxide in depressive and anxiety disorders: II. Efficacy in anxious outpatients. *Arch. Gen. Psychiatry* 43 : 79, 1986.

Nagy, L. M., Krystal, J. H., Woods, S. W., and Charney, D. S. Clinical and medication outcome after short-term alprazolam and behavioral group treatment in panic disorder. *Arch. Gen. Psychiatry* 46 : 993, 1989.

Schweizer, E., Patterson, W., Rickels, K, and Rosenthal, M. Double-blind, placebo-controlled study of once-a-day, sustained-release preparation of alprazolam for the treatment of panic disorder. *Am. J. Psychiatry* 150 : 1210, 1993.

Tesar, G. E., Rosenbaum, J. F., Pollack, M. H., et al. Double-blind, placebo-controlled comparison of clonazepam and alprazolam for panic disorder. *J. Clin. Psychiatry* 52 : 69, 1991.

Depression

Lipman, R. S., Covi, L., Rickels, K., et al. Imipramine and chlordiazepoxide in depressive and anxiety disorders: I. Efficacy in depressed outpatients. *Arch. Gen. Psychiatry* 43 : 68, 1986.

Rickels, K., Chung, H. R., Csanalosi, I. B., et al. Alprazolam, diazepam, imipramine, and placebo in outpatients with major depression. *Arch. Gen. Psychiatry* 44 : 862, 1987.

Insomnia

Dement, W. C. The proper use of sleeping pills in the primary care setting. *J. Clin. Psychiatry* 53(12s) : 50, 1992.

Gillin, J. C., and Byerly, W. F. The diagnosis and management of insomnia. *N. Engl. J. Med.* 332 : 239, 1990.

Gillin, J. C., Spinweber, C. L., and Johnson, L. C. Rebound insomnia: A critical review. *J. Clin. Psychopharmacol.* 9 : 161, 1989.

Morin, C. M., Culbert, J. P., and Schwartz, S. M. Nonpharmacological interventions for insomnia: A meta-analysis of treatment efficacy. *Am. J. Psychiatry* 151 : 1172, 1994.

Alcohol Withdrawal

Saitz R., Mayo-Smith M. F., Robert, M. S. et al. Individualized treatment for alcohol withdrawal: A randomized double-blind controlled Trial. *J.A.M.A.* 272 : 519, 1994.

Clonazepam for Mania

Aronson, T. A., Shukla, S., and Hirschkowitz, J. Clonazepam treatment of five lithium-refractory patients with bipolar disorder. *Am. J. Psychiatry* 146 : 77, 1989.

Sachs, G. A., Rosenbaum, J. F., and Jones, L. Adjunctive clonazepam for maintenance treatment of bipolar disorder. *J. Clin. Psychopharmacol.* 10 : 42, 1990.

Benzodiazepines in Psychotic Disorders

Modell, J. G., Lenox, R. H., and Weiner, S. Inpatient clinical trial of lorazepam for the management of manic agitation. *J. Clin. Psychopharmacol.* 5 : 109, 1985.

Wolkowitz, O. M., and Pickar, D. Benzodiazepines in the treatment of schizophrenia: A review and reappraisal. *Am. J. Psychiatry* 148 : 714, 1991.

Catatonia

Salam, S. A., Pillai, A. K., and Beresford, T. P. Lorazepam for psychogenic catatonia. *Am. J. Psychiatry* 144 : 1082, 1987.

Therapeutic Use

Herman, J. B., Rosenbaum, J. F., and Brotman, A. W. The alprazolam to clonazepam switch for the treatment of panic disorder. *J. Clin. Psychopharmacol.* 7 : 175, 1987.

Uhlenhuth, E. H., DeWit, H., Balter, M. B., et al. Risks and benefits of long-term benzodiazepine use. *J. Clin. Psychopharmacol.* 8 : 161, 1988.

Toxicity

Scharf, M. B., Khosla, N., Brocker, N., and Goff, P. Differential amnestic properties of short- and long-acting benzodiazepines. *J. Clin. Psychiatry* 45 : 51, 1984.

Sunter, J. P., Bal, T. S., and Cowan, W. K. Three cases of fatal triazolam poisoning. *Br. Med. J.* 297 : 719, 1988.

Dependence and Abuse

American Psychiatric Association. *Benzodiazepine Dependence, Toxicity, and Abuse.* Washington, D.C.: American Psychiatric Association, 1990.

Ciraulo, D. A., Barnhill, J. G., Ciraulo, A. M., et al. Parental alcoholism as a risk factor in benzodiazepine abuse: A pilot study. *Am. J. Psychiatry* 146 : 1333, 1989.

Ciraulo, D. A., Sands, B. F., and Shader, R. I. Critical review of liability for benzodiazepine abuse among alcoholics. *Am. J. Psychiatry* 145 : 1501, 1988.

Sellers, E. M., Schneiderman, J. F., Romach, M. K., et al. Comparative drug effects and abuse liability of lorazepam, buspirone, and secobarbital in nondependent subjects. *J. Clin. Psychopharmacol.* 12 : 79, 1992.

Weintraub, M., Singh, S., Byrne, L., et al. Consequences of the 1989 New York State triplicate benzodiazepine prescription regulations. *J.A.M.A.* 266 : 2392, 1991.

Discontinuation

Fyer, A. J., Liebowitz, M. R., Gorman, J. M., et al. Discontinuation of alprazolam treatment in panic patients. *Am. J. Psychiatry* 144 : 303, 1987.

Rickels, K., Case, W. G., Schweizer, E., et al. Long-term benzodiazepine users 3 years after participation in a discontinuation program. *Am. J. Psychiatry* 148 : 757, 1991.

Roy-Byrne, P. P., Dager, S. R., Cowley, D. S., et al. Relapse and rebound following discontinuation of benzodiazepine treatment of panic attacks: Alprazolam versus diazepam. *Am. J. Psychiatry* 146 : 860, 1989.

Use in the Elderly

Ray, W. A., Griffin, M. R., and Downey, W. Benzodiazepines of long and short elimination half-life and the risk of hip fracture. *J.A.M.A.* 262 : 3303, 1989.

Use in Pregnancy

Laegrid, L., Olegard, R., Wahlstrom, J., et al. Abnormalities in children exposed to benzodiazepines in utero. *Lancet* 1 : 108, 1987.

Rosenberg, L., Mitchell, A. A., Parsells, J. L., et al. Lack of relation of oral clefts to diazepam use during pregnancy. *N. Engl. J. Med.* 309 : 1282, 1983.

Buspirone

Grady, T. A., Pigott, T. A., L'Heureux, F., et al. Double-blind study of adjuvant buspirone for fluoxetine-treated patients with obsessive-compulsive disorder. *Am. J. Psychiatry* 150 : 819, 1993.

Kranzler, H. R., Burleson, J. A., Del Boca, F. K., et al. Buspirone treatment of anxious alcoholics. *Arch. Gen. Psychiatry* 51 : 720, 1994.

7

Other Drugs: Psychostimulants, Beta-Adrenergic Blockers, Clonidine, Verapamil, Disulfiram, and Tacrine

PSYCHOSTIMULANTS

A wide variety of compounds (e.g., caffeine and strychnine) can produce central nervous system (CNS) stimulation. However, the stimulant drugs that have found use in psychiatry are sympathomimetic amines, of which the prototype is amphetamine. Amphetamine was first used as a bronchodilator, respiratory stimulant, and analeptic during the 1930s. Psychostimulants were used in the treatment of depression until they were supplanted by tricyclic antidepressants and monoamine oxidase inhibitors (MAOIs) in the 1950s.

The clinical utility of stimulants has been limited by their tendency to cause tolerance and psychological dependence and by their abuse potential. Until recently, large quantities of these drugs were being diverted to nonprescription use, often through the intermediary so-called script doctors who prescribed them without proper indication. In 1970, the Food and Drug Administration (FDA) reclassified these drugs as schedule II, the most restrictive classification for drugs that are medically useful. They are currently approved only for the treatment of attention-deficit/hyperactivity disorder (ADHD) and for narcolepsy. However, they have several other possible uses in psychiatric practice (Table 7-1). Those psychostimulants that are most widely used in clinical practice are dextroamphetamine, methylphenidate, and pemoline (Table 7-2).

Chemistry

Amphetamine is racemic beta-phenylisopropanolamine; dextroamphetamine is the D-isomer, which is 3–4 times more potent than the L-isomer as a CNS stimulant. Methylphenidate is a piperidine derivative that is structurally similar to amphetamine. Pemoline is structurally unrelated (Fig. 7-1).

Pharmacology

Absorption and Metabolism

Amphetamine is well absorbed after oral administration. It has a short half-life (8–12 hours); thus, it is usually administered bid–tid. It crosses the blood-brain barrier easily and develops high concentrations in the brain. Amphetamine is partly metabolized in the liver and partly excreted unchanged in the urine. Its excretion is hastened by acidification of the urine.

Methylphenidate is well absorbed after oral administration. It has a very short biologic life; it reaches peak plasma concentrations in 1–2 hours and has an elimination half-life of 1–2 hours. Clinically, its effects last 3–4 hours, or even less in some patients. Thus multiple doses (3–4) are required during the day. Its concentrations in the brain appear to be higher than those in the blood. Methylphenidate is metabolized by hepatic microsomal enzymes.

Pemoline has a long half-life, permitting once daily dosing. Its therapeutic actions in ADHD are usually delayed by 3–4 weeks.

Table 7-1. Indications for psychostimulants

Effective
  Narcolepsy
  Attention-deficit/hyperactivity disorder (in children)
Probably effective
  Treatment of apathy and withdrawal (in the medically ill and elderly)
  Potentiation of narcotic analgesics
Possibly effective
  Residual attention-deficit disorder (in adults)

Table 7-2. Available preparations

Drug	Trade Name	Dosage Forms
Dextroamphetamine	Dexedrine and generics	5-mg tablets 5-mg/5-ml elixir 5-, 10-, 15-mg SR tablets
Methylphenidate	Ritalin and generics	5-, 10-, 20-mg tablets 20-mg SR tablets
Pemoline	Cylert	18.75-, 37.5-, 75.0-mg tablets

SR = sustained release.

It is 60% metabolized by the liver and 40% excreted unchanged in the urine.

All psychostimulant drugs can compete for hepatic enzymes and thus increase the levels of other drugs. Tolerance to the sympathomimetic effects and to the drug-induced euphoria of amphetamine and methylphenidate develops rapidly. Thus, chronic abusers often take very large doses that would be extremely toxic or lethal if taken by a nontolerant individual.

Mechanism of Action
Amphetamine and the similarly acting methylphenidate are often termed "indirectly acting" amines. This is because they act by causing release of norepinephrine, dopamine, and serotonin from presynaptic nerve terminals as opposed to having direct agonist effects on the postsynaptic receptors themselves. In addition, amphetamine inhibits both norepinephrine and dopamine reuptake and has very mild MAOI effects, thus prolonging and enhancing the effects of the amines it releases from presynaptic terminals.

Amphetamine and its derivatives probably increase alertness by stimulating monoamine release by the ascending reticular activating system. Hypothalamic effects are probably responsible for its appetite suppressant properties. Its stimulatory effects on locomotion and its tendency to produce euphoria are largely a result of facilitation of dopaminergic neurotransmission in the striatum and limbic forebrain. It has been shown in animal models that dopamine lesions or dopamine receptor antagonists block the locomotor stimulant and reinforcing effects of amphetamine, while alpha- and

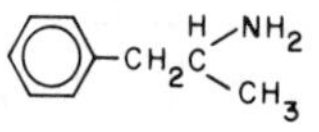

Amphetamine

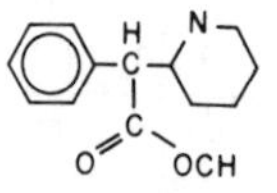

Methylphenidate
(Ritalin)

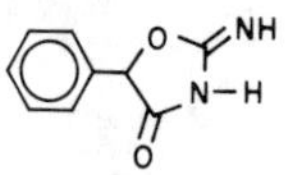

Pemoline
(Cylert)

Fig. 7-1. Chemical structures of psychostimulants.

beta-adrenergic receptor antagonists do not. Amphetamine and its derivatives are potent stimulants of the sympathetic nervous system because they enhance noradrenergic neurotransmission. The peripheral effects of the amphetamine-like drugs at therapeutic doses include mild increases in both systolic and diastolic blood pressure and often a reflex slowing of the heart rate. With higher doses, the heart rate increases and there may be arrhythmias. Pemoline, which is structurally different, has fewer peripheral sympathetic effects than amphetamine.

The mechanism of action of psychostimulants in ADHD is unknown. In contrast to sympathomimetic effects and euphoria, tolerance to the therapeutic effects in ADHD appear to be quite rare. A prior hypothesis held that somehow the stimulants "paradoxically" sedated children with ADHD, but this appears not to be the case because the effects of amphetamine in children with ADHD differ only in degree, not in kind, from its effects in normal children.

Chronic use of high-dose amphetamines and related compounds may produce a psychotic syndrome with prominent paranoid ideation and stereotypic movements. It has been theorized that amphetamine-induced psychosis is caused primarily by the facilitation of dopaminergic neurotransmission in the forebrain.

Therapeutic Indications

Attention-Deficit/Hyperactivity Disorder

The symptoms of this childhood disorder include inattention, impulsiveness, and hyperactivity. Stimulant drugs are an effective treatment in 70–80% of children with ADHD but are best used as part of a comprehensive treatment program. Stimulant drugs improve attention and decrease impulsiveness and hyperactivity. However, they do not help with specific learning disabilities that are often associated with ADHD (e.g., dyslexia). Stimulants are not indicated for "problem children" who do not meet the diagnostic criteria for ADHD.

Methylphenidate is the most commonly used agent, although dextroamphetamine is equally effective. Pemoline also appears to be effective, although its use is less well established. The dosage of dextroamphetamine and methylphenidate is 0.3–1.5 mg/kg/day in divided doses. Pemoline is given at 0.5–3.0 mg/kg/day in a single daily dose. The tricyclic antidepressant desipramine has been used as an alternative to psychostimulants for childhood ADHD, but reports of sudden death in some children treated with desipramine clearly favor the use of psychostimulants as first-line drugs. The antidepressant bupropion, which has stimulant-like properties, and clonidine are currently under study for this indication.

Residual Attention-Deficit Disorder in Adults

DIAGNOSIS. Residual attention-deficit disorder in adulthood is a controversial condition, both diagnostically and therapeutically. The diagnosis requires an established diagnosis of attention-deficit disorder with or without hyperactivity in childhood, with residual inattention and impulsiveness in adulthood. The difficulty in diagnosing and studying this disorder reflects, in part, the difficulty of making a retrospective diagnosis of childhood ADHD based on the memories of the patient, the patient's parents, and teachers. As more children with well-documented ADHD reach adulthood, prospective studies should provide a clearer picture of this putative adult disorder. Another difficulty with the diagnosis is that adults with residual ADHD frequently suffer one or more comorbid psychiatric disorders, most frequently mood, substance abuse, and personality disorders, that may have significant symptom overlap with ADHD.

By themselves, the typical adult "residual symptoms" of ADHD are nonspecific, including restlessness, difficulty in concentrating, excitability, impulsiveness, and irritability. These symptoms often lead to poor job or academic performance, anxiety, temper outbursts, antisocial behavior, and substance abuse.

TREATMENT. According to Wender and associates (1985), 21 of 37 adults with residual ADHD showed moderate to marked symptomatic improvement on methylphenidate (average dose 43.2 mg/day in divided doses, range 10–80), whereas only 4 of 37 adult patients responded to placebo. Pemoline had less clear benefits in a previous study. However, another study (Mattes et al., 1984) that compared adults both with and without a childhood history who had current symptoms consistent with ADHD found that methylphenidate (average dose 48.2 mg/day) helped only a small number of patients (16 of 66) and that a childhood history of ADHD did not predict which of these phenomenologically similar patients would respond. The discrepancies between these studies may be due to the lack of an ADHD-like control population in the study favoring psychostimulant use and the failure to exclude from the negative study patients with additional diagnoses (e.g., depression, personality disorder). Diagnosis and treatment of residual ADHD must still be considered poorly established. Methylphenidate might be administered to adults with ADHD-like symptoms as an empirical trial. The best candidates are patients with a childhood diagnosis of ADHD

Table 7-3.   Dosage range (mg/day)

Drug	Usual Dosage Range	Extreme Dosage Range
Dextroamphetamine	10–30	2.5–60
Methylphenidate	20–40	5.0–80
Pemoline	56.25–75.0	37.5–112.5

whose symptoms include difficulty in concentrating, irritability, impulsiveness, and restlessness. Patients with major depression, borderline or antisocial personality disorder, or a history of drug abuse are probably better treated with other modalities. When effective, the average dosage of methylphenidate is about 40 mg/day given in 3–4 divided doses, but the range may be wide. Dosages above 80 mg/day should generally be avoided. The medication is begun at a low dosage and titrated upward as side effects permit until a therapeutic response is achieved. Anecdotal experience suggests that those who respond for this indication do not develop tolerance (Table 7-3).

Narcolepsy

Narcolepsy is a disorder of excessive daytime sleepiness combined with irresistible sleep attacks of short duration. In addition, patients may suffer from cataplexy, periods of partial or complete loss of motor tone (often precipitated by an episode of strong emotior), sleep paralysis, and/or hypnagogic hallucinations. The symptoms of daytime sleepiness and sleep attacks are most effectively treated with psychostimulants. Unlike use in ADHD, tolerance often develops with some narcoleptics using very high doses of stimulants. The range for both methylphenidate and dextroamphetamine is 20–200 mg/day in divided doses. Alternatively, MAOIs (e.g., phenelzine, 30–75 mg/day) may be successful in treating sleep attacks. Cataplexy does not typically respond to psychostimulants or MAOIs, but it may respond to tricyclic antidepressants (e.g., imipramine, 75–150 mg/day).

Depressed and Apathetic States

MAJOR DEPRESSION. Despite multiple anecdotal reports and uncontrolled studies suggesting that dextroamphetamine, methylphenidate, or pemoline might be effective in the treatment of major depression, controlled studies have been largely negative or uninterpretable. Selective serotonin reuptake inhibitors (SSRIs), cyclic antidepressants, MAOIs, venlafaxine, and bupropion are all clearly preferable. Given the liabilities of the psychostimulants, including the development of tolerance, abuse potential, and side effects such as insomnia, anxiety, and agitation, there is little reason to prescribe these drugs as primary treatments for major depression. For patients who might benefit from stimulant-like effects during the treatment of depression or who have a history of serious weight gain on cyclic antidepressants, bupropion or an SSRI is a better choice than one of the psychostimulants.

Psychostimulants have been used with some success as adjuncts to cyclic antidepressants in the treatment of major depression in situations in which an adequate therapeutic trial of a cyclic antidepressant has not produced a full therapeutic response. For example, methylphenidate, 10–30 mg/day in divided doses, has been added to cyclic antidepressant regimens. Psychostimulants produce a small increase in tricyclic serum levels, but there is no evidence to suggest that this is the mechanism by which patients improve. The use of psychostimulants as adjuncts to tricyclic antidepressants is less well established than the use of other adjuncts such as lithium (see Chap. 3). Psychostimulants might be expected to worsen the common side effects of fluoxetine and other SSRIs (e.g., agitation, insomnia) and must be considered dangerous in combination with MAOIs despite occasional anecdotal reports of their combined use.

APATHETIC AND WITHDRAWN STATES IN MEDICALLY ILL PATIENTS. Medically ill patients (especially the elderly) may develop states of apathy, withdrawal, and a loss of appetite without the full manifestation of a major depressive episode. These states can compromise medical care by decreasing the patient's compliance with treatment and interest in life and diminishing adequate caloric intake. While such patients might respond to antidepressant drugs, the time course of improvement (several weeks) is a definite disadvantage when medical treatment might be compromised. The judicious use of psychostimulants may improve the patient's mood, interest, compliance, and, in some cases, appetite. When effective, the stimulants work rapidly. They produce few side effects; in fact, their cardiovascular side effect profile is safer than that of the tricyclic antidepressants or trazodone. Their major limiting side effects are insomnia (usually controllable by giving doses early in the day), agitation (which requires a dosage decrease or discontinuation), and, very rarely, toxic psychoses.

Although there are many case series and retrospective reports in the literature, this indication for psychostimulants remains to be studied in well-designed trials. Use of psychostimulants should be avoided in patients with a history of stimulant abuse and perhaps in all drug abusers.

When prescribing stimulants to medically ill patients, generally only a short treatment course proves necessary (several days to several weeks) until the precipitating problem has passed. Patients are begun on low dosages (5 mg bid in the elderly, 10 mg bid or tid in younger patients) with gradual increases until a therapeutic effect is achieved.

Potentiation of Narcotic Analgesics

Oral dextroamphetamine can both reduce narcotic requirements in patients who are terminally ill and counteract excess sedation produced by high doses of narcotic drugs. This can be particularly useful in cancer patients who have severe pain requiring high narcotic doses but who object to excessive sedation. Dextroamphetamine, 5–20 mg, has been used successfully either as a single dose early in the day or in divided doses. When dextroamphetamine is added, the narcotic dosage should be decreased slightly.

Obesity

Although psychostimulants were previously used as appetite suppressants in the treatment of obesity, their effect was found to be too short-lived to be of value in most weight reduction programs. Tolerance to the anorectic effect usually develops, severely limiting the usefulness of stimulants for this indication.

Therapeutic Use

Before Starting Psychostimulants

Prior to starting psychostimulants, patients should have a physical examination with attention to heart rate, rhythm, and blood pressure. Psychostimulants should be administered very carefully in patients with hypertension, and attention should be paid to follow-up monitoring. Psychostimulants should probably be withheld from patients with tachyarrhythmias. In children, a neurologic examination should be performed with attention to the presence of tics and dyskinetic movements (stimulants may precipitate or worsen Gilles de la Tourette syndrome and dyskinesias). In the case of pemoline, it is prudent to obtain baseline liver function tests, since liver function abnormalities occasionally develop. Pemoline should be avoided in patients with preexisting liver disease; amphetamine and methylphenidate can be used, but in lower than usual dosages. For patients with renal disease, methylphenidate, which is metabolized by the liver, is the best choice.

Psychostimulant Use

Dextroamphetamine is usually begun at dosages of 5–10 mg bid in adults and at 5 mg qd–bid in children and the elderly. For children under 6 and in debilitated elderly patients, a starting dosage of 2.5 mg qd–bid is prudent. The dosage is increased until the desired therapeutic effects are achieved. In healthy adults, the usual dosage range is 20–30 mg/day, although dosages as high as 60 mg/day may be needed. The dosage for children is 0.3–1.5 mg/kg/day. Detroamphetamine is usually given bid–tid, with the last dose given by late afternoon to avoid insomnia (see Table 7-3).

Methylphenidate is usually begun at 10 mg bid–tid in adults; children and the elderly might be given a test dose of 10 mg and then begun, initially, on 5–10 mg bid. The dosage is slowly increased (10 mg every 2–4 days) until therapeutic results are achieved. The average daily adult dose is 30–40 mg, although doses as high as 80 mg may be used. Dosages for children are 0.3–1.5 mg/kg/day. Methylphenidate is usually given in 3 or 4 daily doses to maintain effectiveness and avoid rebound. The sustained-release form can be given qd or bid, although some clinicians find its action not adequately prolonged.

Pemoline has little established use in adults. For children with ADHD, it is usually begun at 37.5 mg/day and increased weekly by 18.75 mg until a therapeutic effect is achieved. The usual dosage range is 0.5–3.0 mg/kg/day in a single daily dose. Patients given pemoline should have their liver function tests monitored periodically.

Use in Pregnancy

These drugs are lipophilic and thus cross the placental barrier. There appear to be no compelling reasons to use these drugs during pregnancy; thus, they should be avoided.

Use in the Elderly

These drugs are safe in elderly patients but should be used in lower dosages. Generally, dextroamphetamine or methylphenidate is used. Little information exists on the use of pemoline in the elderly.

Side Effects and Toxicity

Central Nervous System Side Effects

The major adverse effects of psychostimulants are central. These include anorexia, insomnia (which can often be minimized by administration early in the day), changes in arousal (either over-stimulated and anxious or alternatively listless and lethargic), and changes in mood (either overly euphoric or occasionally tearful and oversensitive). Dysphoric reactions are more commonly reported in children. Rarely, patients develop toxic psychoses with therapeutic use. High doses, as may occur in some narcoleptics and drug abusers, may produce psychosis with marked paranoia.

Other Side Effects

Patients with underlying fixed or labile hypertension may have mild elevations in blood pressure; rarely, this is severe enough to require discontinuation of the drug. Sinus tachycardia and other tachyar-rhythmias rarely occur at clinical doses. In general, these drugs have greater cardiovascular safety than tricyclic antidepressants. Other side effects include headaches and abdominal pain. Intra-venous amphetamine abusers have developed necrotizing angiitis affecting the brain.

In children, there has been concern about possible long-term growth and weight suppression, although this problem appears to be mild. Children given time off the drug (e.g., during summer vacation) appear to make up any weight loss. Pemoline produces liver function test abnormalities in some patients.

Abuse and Withdrawal

Stimulant Abuse

A major drawback to the use of psychostimulants is their potential for abuse, dependence, and addiction. Amphetamines are abused orally and intravenously, and methylphenidate is abused orally. Pemoline does not appear to be commonly abused. These drugs produce feelings of euphoria and enhanced self-confidence. In the high doses of abuse, there are often signs of adrenergic hyperactivity (i.e., increased pulse and blood pressure, dry mouth, and pupillary dilatation). High doses of amphetamine may result in stereotyped behaviors, bruxism, formication, irritability, restlessness, emotional lability, and paranoia. With chronic abuse, a paranoid psychosis may develop, characterized by paranoid delusions, ideas of reference, and auditory, visual, or tactile hallucinations.

Withdrawal

Although there are no physical withdrawal symptoms, patients who have used high doses for prolonged periods may experience a marked central syndrome, including fatigue, hypersomnia, hyperphagia, and severe depression in the short-term and anhedonia, dysphoria, and drug craving in the long-term. Currently, there is no proven pharmacologic treatment for psychostimulant dependence and with-drawal. Referral to a comprehensive treatment program is usually the best course. Patients should be observed for the emergence of a major depressive syndrome and suicidality or alternatively for recurrent drug abuse.

Overdose

Overdose with psychostimulants results in a syndrome of marked sympathetic hyperactivity (i.e., hypertension, tachycardia, hyperthermia) often accompanied by toxic psychosis or delirium. Patients may be irritable, paranoid, or violent. Grand mal seizures may occur. Death may result from hypertension, hyperthermia, arrhythmias, or uncontrollable seizures.

Treatment consists of supportive care and blockade of adrenergic receptors. If the patient is unconscious or seizing, the airway must be protected. High fevers should be treated with cooling blankets. Seizures can be controlled with an intravenous benzodiazepine, such as lorazepam (1–2 mg) or diazepam (5–10 mg), repeated as necessary.

Delirium or psychosis usually responds to an antipsychotic agent. If the patient is also hypertensive, chlorpromazine has the advantage of blocking both alpha-adrenergic and dopamine receptors. Dosages of 50 mg IM qid are usually adequate, although dosages up to 100 mg qid may be necessary. Otherwise, haloperidol might be a better choice; 5 mg bid will usually suffice. Additional sedation can be provided by benzodiazepines, such as lorazepam, 1–2 mg PO or 1 mg IM, or diazepam, 5–10 mg PO q1–2h prn. Delirium usually clears in 2–3 days, but paranoid psychoses due to long-term high-dose abuse may take longer to clear. Severe hypertension or tachyarrhythmias can usually be treated with propranolol, 1 mg IV q5–10min prn up to a total of 8 mg.

BETA-ADRENERGIC BLOCKERS

Beta-adrenergic blockers (Fig. 7-2) have been used to treat a variety of psychiatric conditions (Table 7-4), although most of these uses are not well studied and none is approved by the FDA. One or more of the beta-adrenergic blockers is approved for the treatment of hypertension, angina, some tachyarrhythmias, symptoms of thyrotoxicosis, glaucoma, and migraine. Four of these agents have been reported on for psychiatric use in the United States: propranolol, metoprolol, nadolol, and atenolol.

Mechanism of Action

Beta-adrenergic blockers in clinical use are competitive antagonists of norepinephrine and epinephrine at beta-adrenergic receptors. Thus, they are peripherally sympatholytic. A detailed understanding of their central actions awaits a more complete description of the functions of norepinephrine in the CNS.

Within the brain, norepinephrine is produced by a small number of neurons, all located in the brainstem tegmentum. The major noradrenergic nucleus is the locus ceruleus, found within the dorsal pons, which projects widely throughout the CNS. Functionally, noradrenergic systems in the brain appear to be involved in modulation of global vigilance, regulation of hormone release, modulation of pain perception, and central regulation of the sympathetic nervous system. It has been hypothesized that noradrenergic systems are involved in important aspects of anxiety and fear. Peripherally, norepinephrine is the major transmitter of postganglionic sympathetic neurons. Epinephrine has only a limited role in the CNS; it appears to be involved in blood pressure control. Peripherally, both epinephrine and norepinephrine are released as stress hormones from the adrenal medulla.

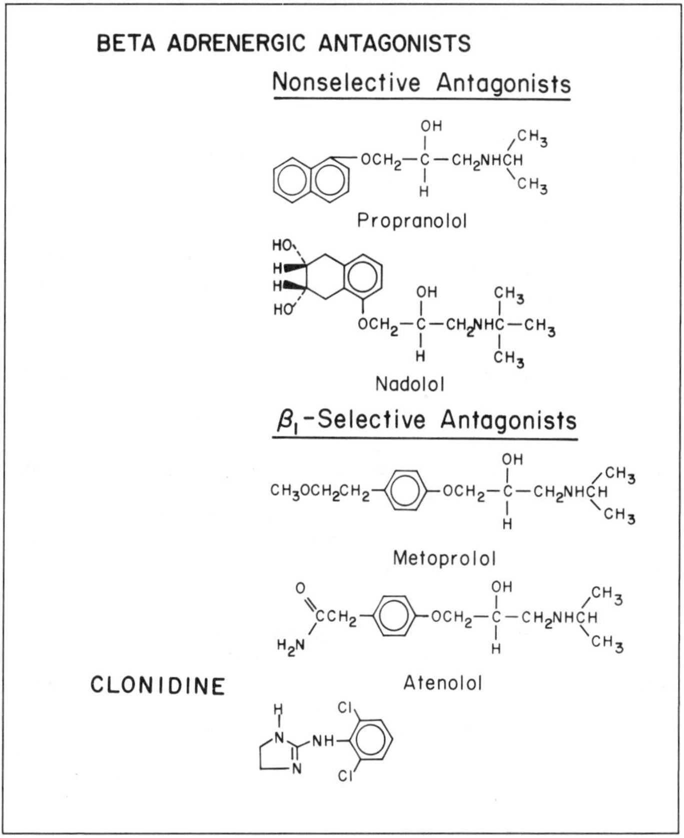

BETA ADRENERGIC ANTAGONISTS
Nonselective Antagonists

Propranolol

Nadolol

β_1-Selective Antagonists

Metoprolol

Atenolol

CLONIDINE

Fig. 7-2. Chemical structures of beta-adrenergic antagonists and clonidine.

Table 7-4. Psychiatric uses for beta-adrenergic receptor antagonists

Effective
  Performance anxiety
  Lithium tremor
  Neuroleptic-induced akathisia

Probably effective
  Adjunct to benzodiazepines in ethanol withdrawal

Possibly effective
  Impulsive violence in patients with organic brain syndromes
  Alternative to benzodiazepines in generalized anxiety disorder

Norepinephrine and epinephrine share two types of receptors, called alpha and beta, each of which has at least two subtypes. Alpha$_1$-receptors are located postsynaptically in both the sympathetic nervous system and the brain. In the brain, alpha$_1$-receptors are found on both neurons and blood vessels. Stimulation of alpha$_1$-receptors produces vasoconstriction. Prazosin is a selective alpha$_1$-receptor antagonist used as an antihypertensive drug; specific alpha$_1$-receptor antagonists are not used in psychiatry at present. Alpha$_2$-receptors are mostly presynaptic autoreceptors (in both sympathetic terminals and locus ceruleus neurons in the brain). Clonidine is a selective agonist at alpha$_2$-adrenergic receptors; yohimbine is a selective antagonist. Since alpha$_2$-receptors function, in large part, as inhibitory autoreceptors on noradrenergic neurons, clonidine decreases central noradrenergic neurotransmission, thereby producing centrally mediated hypotension and other effects.

Beta$_1$-receptors are found in the brain and heart. They stimulate the heart both chronotropically and inotropically. Metoprolol, atenolol, and practolol are selective beta$_1$-receptor antagonists. Beta$_2$-receptors are found in the brain on glial cells more than on neurons; peripherally, they are found in the lung and blood vessels. Stimulation of beta$_2$-receptors produces bronchodilation and vasodilation. Salbutamol and terbutaline are selective agonists used clinically in the treatment of asthma. No obvious clinical use for selective beta$_2$-receptor antagonists exists.

Pharmacology

Four major features differentiate the beta-blockers: their relative receptor selectivity, their relative lipophilicity, their route of metabolism, and their half-lives. The advent of relatively selective beta-receptor antagonists (metoprolol and atenolol), with less effect at beta$_2$- than beta$_1$-receptors, has decreased the problem of bronchospasm induced by the older nonselective drugs. The selectivity is only relative, however; caution must still be exercised in treating patients with asthma. Both nonselective and beta$_1$-selective compounds have been used for psychiatric disorders.

Beta-receptor blockers differ markedly in their lipophilicity. The least lipophilic drugs, nadolol and atenolol, cross the blood-brain barrier poorly and therefore have a higher ratio of peripheral to central effects, while the more lipophilic drugs, propranolol and metoprolol, have potent central as well as peripheral effects. Compounds of intermediate lipophilicity include acebutolol and timolol. Pindolol is also of intermediate lipophilicity; however, it differs from the other beta-blockers because it has intrinsic sympathomimetic activity also. Pindolol has no current use in psychiatry.

The drugs also vary markedly in elimination half-life. Nadolol and atenolol have relatively long half-lives, thus allowing once a day administration. In contrast, propranolol requires multiple daily dosing unless a sustained-release form is used. The major features of commonly used beta-adrenergic blockers are given in Table 7-5.

The beta-blockers do not appear to induce tolerance to their psychiatric effects or to have abuse potential.

Psychiatric Use

Performance Anxiety

Performance anxiety, a well-known example of which is "stage fright," is considered to be a form of social phobia. When severe,

Table 7-5.   Relevant pharmacologic properties of commonly used beta-adrenergic blockers

Drug	Selectivity	Lipophilicity	Half-life (hr)	Route of Elimination
Propranolol	None	High	3–6	Hepatic
Metoprolol	Beta$_1$	High	3–4	Hepatic
Atenolol	Beta$_1$	Low	6–9	Renal
Nadolol	None	Low	14–24	Renal

performance anxiety can interfere with life activities that are important to many individuals. It may lead to poor performance in or avoidance of such activities as interviews, speaking in class, public speaking, acting, or music. Symptoms include dry mouth, hoarse voice, pounding heart, difficulty in breathing, tremor, and, occasionally, weakness and dizziness. The anxiety may feed on itself, creating a vicious cycle of anticipatory anxiety leading up to the activity and worsening anxiety during the activity. When this syndrome interferes with important activities, treatment is indicated. Beta-blockers, used in optimal doses, have minimal central side effects and generally improve performance. Benzodiazepines, on the other hand, which may cause some sedation or disinhibition, are likely to worsen performance.

A single dose of propranolol, 10–40 mg or the equivalent, usually suffices. The dose can be given 20–30 minutes prior to the anxiogenic event. It is reasonable to administer a test dose on some anxiogenic occasion prior to an all-important engagement. Since most of the troublesome symptoms are peripheral, less lipophilic agents (e.g., nadolol or atenolol) are also effective. Cognitive/behavior therapies are alternatives for individuals who do not wish to take or do not tolerate beta-blockers.

Lithium Tremor

Lithium may cause an action tremor even when used at therapeutic (nontoxic) blood levels. While new onset or coarsening of tremor suggests lithium toxicity, a stable tremor occurring at therapeutic blood levels may be troublesome and merit treatment. Several interventions can be tried. First, it is important to establish that the patient is on the lowest dosage therapeutic for that individual. Second, it is helpful if the patient minimizes or eliminates caffeine consumption. Third, for some patients, dosing can be altered so that the entire dose is taken at bedtime (see Chap. 4); using such a dosage regimen, peak levels (which are most likely to cause tremor) occur during the night. Finally, if the patient is still bothered by tremor, especially if it interferes with daily activities, beta-blockers can be administered. Propranolol is often helpful in the range of 20–160 mg/day or the equivalent given in 2 or 3 divided doses. Less lipophilic drugs (i.e., atenolol or nadolol) may also be effective for this indication.

Neuroleptic-Induced Akathisia

This serious side effect of antipsychotic drugs is fully described in Chapter 2. Some clinicians believe that beta-adrenergic blockers are the most effective treatment for neuroleptic-induced akathisia, and in at least one study, they were shown to be superior to benzodiazepines. For refractory akathisia, or akathisia occurring with parkinsonian symptoms, beta-blockers or benzodiazepines can be given in combination with an anticholinergic drug.

In case reports and small studies, patients have responded to both propranolol and nadolol. Dosages of propranolol were in the range of 30–80 mg/day in divided doses; dosages of nadolol ranged from 40–80 mg/day given as a single dose. Propranolol worked rapidly once an effective dosage was found; it had no effect on other extrapyramidal symptoms.

Adjunct to Benzodiazepines in Ethanol Withdrawal

In a randomized double-blind trial (Kraus et al., 1985), atenolol was found to be a useful adjunct to (not a replacement for) benzodiazepines in ethanol withdrawal. Sixty-one patients received atenolol, and 59 received placebo. Atenolol was administered as follows: no drug if the heart rate was less than 50, 50 mg if it was 50–79, and 100 mg for a heart rate of 80 or above. The drug was given once a day. Compared with those on placebo, the vital signs and tremors of patients on atenolol improved more rapidly from the first day, and shorter hospital stays and fewer benzodiazepines were required. Since beta-blockers do not cross-react with ethanol, they are probably not an adequate single agent for detoxification.

Violent Outbursts in Patients with Organic Brain Syndromes

Both case reports and small controlled trials have suggested utility for beta-adrenergic blockers in the treatment of violent outbursts, especially in patients with organic brain syndromes. Patients who have been the subjects of reports have ranged in neurologic impairment from slight to very severe. Propranolol, in dosages of 40–520 mg/day in 2–4 divided doses, has been reported to be effective; nadolol, 120 mg, has been reported to be superior to placebo. In many case series, patients were being treated concomitantly with other drugs, including antipsychotics, carbamazepine, and lithium, which had not, by themselves, curbed the violent outbursts. Further study is needed, but a careful empirical clinical trial of a beta-adrenergic blocker could reasonably be undertaken in patients with organic brain syndromes with episodic violence refractory to nonpharmacologic measures, so long as cardiovascular and respiratory status are well monitored and objective records of the frequency and severity of violent outbursts are maintained. Although doses of propranolol above 200 mg/day have been reported, they are not recommended.

Generalized Anxiety and Panic Disorder

Multiple controlled trials suggest that although the beta-adrenergic blockers are effective in treating autonomic symptoms associated with generalized anxiety and panic attacks, they are less effective than other agents (e.g., benzodiazepines in generalized anxiety or antidepressants in panic disorder) in treating the psychological aspects of anxiety and in overall outcome. When used for generalized anxiety, variable success has been reported with propranolol in dosages of 40–320 mg/day given in 2 or 3 divided doses. The usefulness of beta-blockers in any given patient is empirical. It is important to watch for emergent signs of depression and to discontinue the beta-blocker if depression develops during the course of treatment.

Other Disorders

Very high doses of propranolol have been tried in **schizophrenia** without convincing benefit. Beta-blockers have also been tried in the treatment of **tardive dyskinesia,** also without sustained or reproducible benefit.

Therapeutic Use

Choice of Drug

For patients with asthma or other obstructive pulmonary disorders, a relatively selective $beta_1$-antagonist (metoprolol or atenolol) is preferable. However, for such patients, the risk, even with selective agents, probably outweighs their established psychiatric benefits. Beta-blockers should be used cautiously in diabetics prone to hypoglycemia, since they may interfere with the normal response to hypoglycemia.

For disorders in which a primarily peripheral effect is required and repetitive dosing is expected (lithium tremor), a less lipophilic agent might be chosen (nadolol or atenolol) to minimize potential central side effects (lassitude, depression, sleep disorder). For disorders in which a central effect is desired (e.g., control of violence), more lipophilic agents (propranolol, metoprolol) should be selected.

Use of Beta-Blockers for Psychiatric Disorders

Beta-blockers are begun at low doses, and side effects, such as bradycardia, hypotension, or bronchospasm, should be monitored. Doses are typically withheld if blood pressure is less than 90/60 mm Hg or heart rate is less than 55. Bradycardia or hypotension also precludes dosage increases. If patients develop asthma during treatment for psychiatric symptoms, the dangers of drug therapy may outweigh the established benefits; thus drug discontinuation should be considered.

Propranolol may be started at dosages of 10 mg tid or 10–20 mg bid and slowly increased (e.g., by no more than 20–30 mg/day at first) until therapeutic effects are achieved. It must be given in divided doses because of its short half-life. Metoprolol is usually begun at dosages of 50 mg bid. Nadolol and atenolol can be given in single daily doses.

Patients who have coronary artery disease or hypertension risk rebound worsening when beta-blockers are discontinued; in such patients, slow weaning with careful follow-up is the safest course.

Side Effects and Drug Interactions

Beta-adrenergic blockers have a variety of significant side effects (Table 7-6). Beta-blockers have no apparent effect on memory. They may actually improve performance of tasks that require a mixture of perceptual motor, learning, and memory skills, perhaps because such tasks are sensitive to even low levels of anxiety. Several drug interactions have been reported, including increased levels of theophylline and thyroxine.

CLONIDINE

Although clonidine's primary use is as an antihypertensive drug, it also has properties that make it useful in psychiatric drug therapy. Its principal mechanism of action appears to be as an agonist at $alpha_2$-adrenergic receptors in the CNS. Since the predominant role

Table 7-6. Side effects and toxicity of beta-blockers

Cardiovascular
  Hypotension
  Bradycardia
  Dizziness
  Congestive failure (in patients with compromised myocardial function)
Respiratory
  Asthma (less risk with beta$_1$ selective drugs)
Metabolic
  Worsened hypoglycemia in diabetics on insulin or oral agents
Gastrointestinal
  Nausea
  Diarrhea
  Abdominal pain
Sexual function
  Impotence
Neuropsychiatric
  Lassitude
  Fatigue
  Dysphoria
  Insomnia
  Vivid nightmares
  Depression
  Psychosis (rare)
Other (rare)
  Raynaud's phenomenon
  Peyronie's disease
Withdrawal syndrome
  Rebound worsening of preexisting angina pectoris when beta-blockers
    are discontinued

of central alpha$_2$-receptors is to act as autoreceptors with a negative feedback function, the major effect of clonidine is to decrease the activity of central noradrenergic neurons. This has complex effects, including decreased sympathetic outflow.

The psychiatric uses of clonidine (Table 7-7) are currently experimental. The similarly acting agents guanabenz and guanfacine have rarely been reported on for psychiatric indications.

Clonidine is available for oral use only under the trade name Catapres. Tablets are available in 0.1-, 0.2-, and 0.3-mg strengths.

Pharmacology

Clonidine is almost completely absorbed after oral administration; it achieves peak plasma concentrations in 1–3 hours. The drug is very lipophilic, easily penetrating the blood-brain barrier. Approximately half is metabolized in the liver, and the rest is excreted unchanged by the kidney. It has no known active metabolites. It has an elimination half-life of 9 hours; thus, it is usually given in 2 daily doses.

Psychiatric Use

Opioid Withdrawal

Several controlled trials have demonstrated the usefulness of clonidine during withdrawal from narcotics. Clonidine may suppress

Table 7-7. Uses of clonidine in psychiatry

Probably effective
    Opioid withdrawal
    Gilles de la Tourette syndrome
Investigational
    Mania
    Anxiety disorders
    Neuroleptic-induced akathisia
    Attention deficit hyperactivity disorder (ADHD)

many signs and symptoms of withdrawal, thus enhancing patient comfort and compliance. It is particularly effective in suppressing autonomic symptoms, having proved more effective than morphine or placebo. It is less effective than morphine, however, in treating subjective symptoms of abstinence such as drug craving. Sedation and hypotension limit its usefulness in outpatients.

The mainstay of opiate detoxification is the long-acting opiate methadone. In typical detoxification protocols, the requirement for methadone is determined using objective criteria (hypertension or tachycardia above baseline, dilated pupils, sweating, gooseflesh, rhinorrhea, or lacrimation) rather than subjective complaints. Methadone is administered in dosages of 10 mg PO q4h when at least two objective criteria for withdrawal are met. The total dose of methadone given on day 1 is given the next day in 2 divided doses. Methadone is then withdrawn by 5 mg/day. During the withdrawal of methadone, clonidine may be administered beginning at low dosages, such as 0.1 mg bid or tid, and increased as needed and tolerated. Dosages above 0.3 mg tid are rarely necessary. With completion of withdrawal, clonidine can be rapidly tapered. In neonates with narcotic abstinence syndrome, dosages of 3–4 μg/kg/day have been reported to be quite effective without toxicity.

Withdrawal from Other Drugs

In one small but well-designed study, clonidine was ineffective in treating withdrawal from either long or short half-life benzodiazepines. After an initial report claimed that clonidine aided in cessation of tobacco smoking, a well-designed study found it to be of no benefit.

Gilles de la Tourette Syndrome

This disorder is characterized by multiple motor and phonic tics, which develop during childhood and are chronic in duration. The nature and severity of the symptoms vary markedly among individuals and for any given patient over time. In addition to their motor and phonic symptoms, patients may have difficulty in concentrating, impulsiveness, and obsessions and compulsions.

When severe, this disorder is socially disabling and merits a trial of drug treatment. Although antipsychotic drugs (especially haloperidol and more recently pimozide) have traditionally been used to treat Gilles de la Tourette syndrome (see Chap. 2), clonidine appears to be useful as an alternative. The mechanism by which clonidine is effective in this disorder is unknown. When effective, it may take 2–3 months for its beneficial effects to manifest. In one randomized trial, clonidine, 3–5 μg/kg/day, was superior to placebo in decreasing tic severity. When given for this disorder, clonidine is begun at very low dosages, typically 0.05 mg/day, and slowly titrated upward over several weeks to the range of 0.15–0.3 mg/day given in 2 divided doses. Dosages above 0.5 mg/day often have more side effects than patients are willing to tolerate for the amount of benefit.

Mania

There are case reports and uncontrolled trials suggesting possible efficacy for clonidine in acute mania. Patients in these reports were treated with clonidine alone or in combination with lithium or car-bamazepine. The reported dosages of clonidine were 0.2–0.4 mg bid. Patients were reported to improve within 2–3 days after an effective dosage of clonidine was reached. However, in a double-blind cross-over study of 24 patients with mania, lithium was found to be clearly more effective than clonidine. Evidence for the effectiveness of clonidine in mania or bipolar prophylaxis is unconvincing.

Anxiety Disorders

There have been sporadic reports of effectiveness in panic disorder and generalized anxiety. Although some individuals may benefit, clonidine does not appear to be generally effective.

Neuroleptic-Induced Akathisia

Akathisia, a serious side effect of antipsychotic drugs, is fully dis-cussed in Chapter 2. Clonidine has been reported to help some patients. In both open- and single-blind studies, clonidine in dosages of 0.15–2.0 mg/day (extreme range reported 0.1–0.8 mg/day) in divided doses has a significant effect on both subjective symptoms and objective signs of akathisia. Therapy is limited, however, by sedation and hypotension. Hypotensive side effects may be exacer-bated with concomitant administration of low-potency neuroleptics. Because its efficacy has been less well studied than other drugs and because of these side effects, it is reasonable to reserve the use of clonidine for patients whose akathisia does not respond to anti-psychotic dosage reduction and treatment with anticholinergic drugs, beta-blockers, or benzodiazepines.

Therapeutic Use

Clonidine is begun at low dosages to minimize side effects such as sedation and hypotension. Typically 0.1 mg bid is safe, although in children with Gilles de la Tourette syndrome, the starting dosage may be as low as 0.05 mg/day. The dosage is increased slowly, by no more than 0.1 mg/day, until the desired therapeutic effects are achieved. For most psychiatric uses, optimal dosages are unknown. One group reports that dosages of 5 µg/kg/day in divided doses is effective in opiate withdrawal. Clonidine's maximal effect on blood pressure appears to be at dosages in the range of 0.3 mg bid. In a minority of cases in which clonidine is used as an antihypertensive agent, tolerance occurs; the occurrence of tolerance for psychiatric indications is unknown. Long-term uses in which tolerance might be a problem are in the treatment of akathisia and Gilles de la Tourette syndrome.

Drug Discontinuation

In treating hypertensive patients, sudden withdrawal of clonidine occasionally precipitates a hypertensive crisis that may be life-threatening. This has usually been reported after use of higher dosages, although dosages as low as 0.6 mg/day have been implicated. This hypertensive rebound begins 18–20 hours after the last dose. When rebound hypertension is severe, treatment includes combined alpha- and beta-adrenergic blockers and/or sodium nitroprusside. Because of this possibility, clonidine should be used with care in hypertensive patients, even if the indications for use are psychiatric. It is prudent to wean the drug rather than discontinue it at once in all patients who have received high doses for more than 2–3 weeks.

Side Effects and Toxicity

Almost all of the experience with clonidine comes from patients using it for hypertension, but the side effects in psychiatric patients are likely to be similar. About 50% of patients report dry mouth and some degree of sedation during the first 2–4 weeks of therapy. Tolerance to these effects usually occurs. About 10% of patients discontinue this agent because of persistent side effects, including sedation, postural dizziness, dry mouth or dry eyes, nausea, and impotence. Fluid retention may occur, but this effect is correctable with diuretics.

Central nervous system side effects are particularly important in psychiatric patients because they may be confused with the underlying disorder for which the agent was prescribed. They include

Sedation, drowsiness
Vivid dreams or nightmares
Insomnia
Restlessness
Anxiety
Depression
Visual or auditory hallucinations (rare)

Rare **idiosyncratic side effects** include rash, pruritus, alopecia, hyperglycemia, gynecomastia, and increased sensitivity to alcohol.

Drug interactions are uncommon, but concurrent use with a tricyclic antidepressant may reduce the antihypertensive effect of clonidine.

Overdoses may result in decreased blood pressure, heart rate, and respiratory rate. Patients may be stuporous or comatose with small pupils, thus mimicking an opioid overdose. Treatment consists of ventilatory support, intravenous fluids or pressors for hypotension, and atropine for bradycardia.

VERAPAMIL

Verapamil is a calcium channel blocker primarily used in the treatment of supraventricular tachyarrhythmias and other cardiovascular symptoms. Although some calcium channel antagonists are anticonvulsant, verapamil lacks potent anticonvulsant effects. Several case reports and small studies found it to be effective in the treatment of mania in dosages of 160–480 mg/day (usually divided into 2 daily doses). However, there are also negative reports and studies. In clinical practice, verapamil has not proved particularly useful in the treatment of mania or in bipolar prophylaxis compared with other treatments. Additional, better designed studies are warranted. The main side effects of verapamil are constipation, headache, vertigo, hypotension, and atrioventricular conduction disturbances.

DISULFIRAM

One strategy in the treatment of alcoholism is the use of sensitizing agents that produce a feeling of sickness when the patient consumes ethanol. The rationale behind their use is that the threat of an aversive reaction will deter alcohol consumption. Disulfiram is one of several compounds that can cause sensitization to alcohol, but it is the only one commonly used in the United States. Although controlled clinical trials do not favor the use of sensitizing agents as effective treatments for alcoholism, disulfiram continues to be prescribed in the United States.

Controlled trials (Fuller and Roth, 1979; Fuller et al., 1986) do not indicate any advantage of disulfiram over placebo in achieving total abstinence, in delaying resumption of drinking, or in improving employment status or social stability. At dosages of 250 mg/day, however, the drug appears to increase the proportion of days in which no alcohol is consumed. This modest benefit may decrease the medical complications of alcoholism in the long run, but this has not been proved definitively.

Although disulfiram has only limited value in the general population, some clinicians believe that the drug is useful for selected individuals who remain employed and socially stable. Since these patients have the best outcomes in any case, it is unclear that disulfiram actually contributes to therapeutic success.

Pharmacology and Mechanism of Action

Disulfiram is 80–90% absorbed after an oral dose. Although it has a short half-life (because it is rapidly metabolized by the liver), its biologic effect is long-lived because it is an irreversible inhibitor of certain enzymes, most importantly, aldehyde dehydrogenase. This is a hepatic enzyme involved in the intermediary metabolism of ethanol. In normal ethanol metabolism, acetaldehyde is produced but does not accumulate because it is rapidly oxidized by aldehyde dehydrogenase. However, when this enzyme has been inhibited by disulfiram, acetaldehyde levels accumulate to 5–10 times higher than usual. It is acetaldehyde that is responsible for most of the resulting symptoms.

Disulfiram inhibits enzymes other than aldehyde dehydrogenase. It inhibits hepatic microsomal enzymes, thus interfering with the metabolism of a variety of drugs, including

Phenytoin
Isoniazid
Warfarin
Rifampin
Barbiturates
Long-acting benzodiazepines (e.g., diazepam, chlordiazepoxide)

Disulfiram also inhibits dopamine beta-hydroxylase, thus potentially decreasing the concentrations of norepinephrine and epinephrine in the sympathetic nervous system. This may be partly responsible for the severity of hypotension observed in the disulfiram-alcohol reaction.

The Disulfiram-Alcohol Reaction

Five to ten minutes after consuming alcohol, the patient on disulfiram develops a feeling of heat in the face, followed by facial and then whole body flushing due to vasodilation. This is accompanied by throbbing in the head and neck and a severe headache. Sweating, dry mouth, nausea, vomiting, dizziness, and weakness usually occur. In more severe reactions, there may be chest pain, dyspnea, severe hypotension, and confusion. Death has been reported—usually in patients who have taken more than 500 mg of disulfiram, but occasionally with lower doses. After the symptoms pass, the patient is usually exhausted and often sleeps, after which the patient usually recovers entirely. The symptoms last from 30 minutes to 2 hours. The length and severity depend both on the dose of disulfiram and the amount of ethanol consumed. The threshold for the reaction is approximately 7 ml of 100% ethanol or its equivalent. After a dose of disulfiram, sensitization to ethanol lasts for 6–14 days, the time required to synthesize an adequate number of new molecules of aldehyde dehydrogenase.

Diphenhydramine, 50 mg IM or IV, has been reported to be symptomatically helpful. Severe reactions may require emergency supportive treatment, most often with intravenous fluids for hypotension and dehydration. Shock, requiring pressors, may occur, as may arrhythmias. Respiratory distress often improves with the administration of oxygen.

Therapeutic Use

Disulfiram should only be prescribed to alcoholics who seek total abstinence, agree to use the drug, and appear able to comply with its use. Its use is therefore not recommended in severely impulsive, psychotic, or suicidal patients. In addition, patients should have no medical contraindications to its use. These contraindications include

Pregnancy
Moderate to severe hepatic dysfunction
Renal failure
Peripheral neuropathies
Cardiac disease

Patients must be made to understand the dangers of drinking alcohol while on the drug. They should be warned to avoid ethanol in any form, including such disguised forms as sauces, cough syrups, and even topical preparations such as aftershave.

There is no evidence that disulfiram or any alcohol sensitizing agent is effective long-term (months to years). In individual patients, the agent may be useful as an adjunct to a comprehensive psychosocial treatment plan in which the maintenance of complete abstinence is sought.

Patients should be thoroughly detoxified before starting the drug. The usual dosage is 250 mg qd, usually taken in the morning, when the resolve to remain abstinent is often greatest. Patients who feel drowsy on the drug may prefer to take their dose at bedtime. An optimal dosage that is both safe and effective is not known. Dosages above 250 mg are associated with more severe side effects and do not appear to be warranted. Dosages as low as 100 mg have been used when side effects do not permit higher doses.

Once therapy is established, it is important to assess compliance at regular intervals. A complete blood count and liver function test should be checked every 3–6 months. Disulfiram may be teratogenic and should not be used by pregnant women.

Side Effects and Toxicity

The most common adverse effects are fatigue and drowsiness, which can be managed by taking the dose at bedtime or reducing the dosage. Some patients complain of body odor or halitosis, which also may improve with dosage reduction. Other reported side effects include tremor, headache, impotence, dizziness, and a foul taste in the mouth. Rare but severe side effects include hepatotoxicity and neuropathies. Psychiatric side effects appear to be very rare, although psychosis and catatonic-like reactions have been reported.

A reported overdose of disulfiram alone caused delirium with prominent hallucinations, tachycardia, and hypertension. The patient recovered in 7 days with supportive care plus haloperidol to control delirium.

Drug Interactions

Because hepatic microsomal enzymes are inhibited by disulfiram, levels of several drugs (i.e., vasodilators, alpha- or beta-adrenergic antagonists, antidepressants, antipsychotic agents) may be increased with a risk of toxicity. Hepatic glucuronic acid conjugation is not affected; thus the metabolism of such drugs as oxazepam and lorazepam is not affected.

Certain drugs increase the severity of the disulfiram-alcohol reaction, and their use should be considered as a relative contraindication for disulfiram. The following drugs may worsen the disulfiram-alcohol reaction:

MAOIs
Vasodilators
Alpha- or beta-adrenergic antagonists
Tricyclic antidepressants
Antipsychotic drugs

TACRINE

Tacrine is an acridinamine derivative that has been approved for the treatment of cognitive deficits due to Alzheimer's disease. It is a noncompetitive, reversible inhibitor of acetylcholinesterase.

Pharmacology

Tacrine is highly lipid-soluble, unlike many acetylcholinesterase inhibitors; thus it produces high levels in the brain. Oral absorption produces highly variable plasma levels, which peak at approximately 2 hours after administration. The drug is extensively metabolized in the liver; its half-life is prolonged in the elderly and in individuals with liver disease. In healthy volunteers the elimination half-life is 2 hours; in the elderly it is approximately 3.5 hours.

Mechanism of Action

Alzheimer's disease produces widespread death of neurons in the brain. Cholinergic neurons in the basal forebrain that innervate the cerebral cortex and hippocampus are thought to play critical roles in memory function. In Alzheimer's disease, these cholinergic neurons are often particularly seriously affected. By inhibiting the metabolism of acetylcholine in the brain, tacrine is thought to ameliorate the partial depletion of this neurotransmitter brought about by the dropout of cholinergic neurons. Because Alzheimer's disease is a progressive disease of cell death, tacrine is meant only as a palliative symptomatic treatment for the earlier stages of illness. Because acetylcholine is only one of many neurotransmitters affected, tacrine is only a partial palliative.

Clinical Use

Double-blind placebo-controlled trials of tacrine have demonstrated benefit in a minority of mildly to moderately impaired patients with probable Alzheimer's disease. The study reporting the greatest benefit used high dosages of 160 mg/day, but not all patients in the study could tolerate that dosage. Even for those who respond to tacrine, the benefit is modest, consisting of slower decline or some improvement in cognitive and living skills test scores. There are no data to suggest that tacrine produces clinically significant functional improvement.

Tacrine is usually begun at a dosage of 10 mg qid and is very slowly increased as side effects allow. The maximum dosage is 40 mg qid. Because of hepatic toxicity, aminotransferase activity should be monitored throughout treatment; the manufacturer recommends monitoring weekly.

Adverse Effects and Drug Interactions

Approximately 50% of patients on tacrine develop elevations in hepatic aminotransferase activity. In short-term studies of tacrine, these elevations have usually returned to normal within 6 weeks of drug discontinuation. Approximately 25% of patients studied have had marked abnormalities (at least 3 times the upper limit of normal). Several patients on dosages of 100–200 mg/day have had biopsy-proven hepatitis, which resolved clinically upon drug discontinuation. Other side effects include nausea, vomiting, diarrhea, headache, and ataxia.

Tacrine may interact with drugs metabolized by the hepatic P450 pathway; it has been shown to increase levels of theophylline.

BIBLIOGRAPHY

Psychostimulants

Review

Chiarello, R. J., and Cole, J. O. The use of psychostimulants in general psychiatry. *Arch. Gen. Psychiatry* 44 : 286, 1987.

Therapeutic Indications

Forrest, W. H., Jr., Brown, B. W., Jr., Brown, C. R., et al. Dextroamphetamine with morphine for the treatment of postoperative pain. *N. Engl. J. Med.* 296 : 712, 1977.

Katon, W., and Raskind, M. Treatment of depression in the medically ill elderly with methylphenidate. *Am. J. Psychiatry* 137 : 963, 1980.

Kaufmann, M. W., Marray, G. B., and Cassem, N. H. Use of psychostimulants in medically ill depressed patients. *Psychosomatics* 23 : 817, 1982.

Mannuzza, S., Klein, R. G., Bessler, A., et al. Adult outcome of hyperactive boys: Educational achievement, occupational rank, and psychiatric status. *Arch. Gen. Psychiatry* 50 : 885, 1993.

Mattes, J. A., Boswell, L., and Oliver, H. Methylphenidate effects on symptoms of attention deficit disorder in adults. *Arch. Gen. Psychiatry* 41 : 1059, 1984.

Wender, P. H., Reimherr, F. W., and Wood, D. R. Attention deficit disorder ("minimal brain dysfunction") in adults. *Arch. Gen. Psychiatry* 38 : 449, 1981.

Wender, P. H., Reimherr, F. W., Wood, D., and Ward, M. A controlled study of methylphenidate in the treatment of attention deficit disorder, residual type, in adults. *Am. J. Psychiatry* 142 : 547, 1985.

Wood, D. R., Reimherr, F. W., Wender, P. H., et al. Diagnosis and treatment of minimal brain dysfunction in adults: A preliminary report. *Arch. Gen. Psychiatry* 33 : 1453, 1976.

Beta-adrenergic Blockers

Treatment of Anxiety

James, I., Pearson, R., Griffith, D., et al. Effect of oxprenolol on stage fright in musicians. *Lancet* 2 : 952, 1977.

Kathol, R., Noyes, R., Jr., Slymen, D. J., et al. Propranolol in chronic anxiety disorders: A controlled study. *Arch. Gen. Psychiatry* 37 : 1361, 1981.

Treatment of Aggressive Outbursts

Greendyke, R. M., Schuster, D. B., and Wooton, J. A. Propranolol in the treatment of assaultive patients with organic brain disease. *J. Clin. Psychopharmacol.* 4 : 282, 1984.

Mattes, J. A. Metoprolol for intermittent explosive disorder. *Am. J. Psychiatry* 142 : 1108, 1985.

Ratey, J. J., Morrill, R., and Oxenkrug, G. Use of propranolol for provoked and unprovoked episodes of rage. *Am. J. Psychiatry* 140 : 1356, 1983.

Ratey, J. J., Sorgi, P., O'Driscoll, G. A., et al. Nadolol to treat aggression and psychiatric symptomatology in chronic psychiatric inpatients: A double-blind, placebo-controlled study. *J. Clin. Psychiatry* 53 : 41, 1992.

Treatment of Akathisia

Lipinski, J. F., Zubenko, G. S., Cohen, B. M., and Barreira, P. J. Propranolol in the treatment of neuroleptic-induced akathisia. *Am. J. Psychiatry* 141 : 412, 1984.

Ratey, J. J., Sorgi, P., and Polakoff, S. Nadolol as a treatment for akathisia. *Am. J. Psychiatry* 142 : 640, 1985.

Treatment of Ethanol Withdrawal

Kraus, M. L., Gottlieb, L. D., Horwitz, R. I., and Anscher, M. Randomized clinical trial of atenolol in patients with alcohol withdrawal. *N. Engl. J. Med.* 313 : 905, 1985.

Adverse Effects

Dimsdale, J. E., Newton, R. P., and Joist, T. Neuropsychological side effects of beta-blockers. *Arch. Intern. Med.* 149 : 514, 1989.

Griffin, S. J. and Friedman, M. J. Depressive symptoms in propranolol users. *J. Clin. Psychiatry* 47 : 453, 1986.

Clonidine

Adler, L. A., Angrist, B., Peselow, E., et al. Clonidine in neuroleptic-induced akathisia. *Am. J. Psychiatry* 144 : 235, 1987.

Bond, W. S. Psychiatric indications for clonidine: The neuropharmacologic and clinical basis. *J. Clin. Psychopharmacol.* 6 : 81, 1986.

Cohen, D. J., Detlor J., Young, J. G., et al. Clonidine ameliorates Gilles de la Tourette syndrome. *Arch. Gen. Psychiatry* 37 : 1350, 1980.

Franks, P., Harp, J., and Bell, B. Randomized, controlled trial of clonidine for smoking cessation in a primary care setting. *J.A.M.A.* 262 : 3011, 1989.

Giannini, A. J., Pascarzi, G. A., Loiselle, R. H., et al. Comparison of clonidine and lithium in the treatment of mania. *Am. J. Psychiatry* 143 : 1608, 1986.

Goodman, W. K., Charney, D. S., Price, L. H., et al. Ineffectiveness of clonidine in the treatment of the benzodiazepine withdrawal syndrome: Report of three cases. *Am. J. Psychiatry* 143 : 900, 1986.

Hardy, M. D., Lecrubien, Y., and Widlocher, D. Efficacy of clonidine in 24 patients with acute mania. *Am. J. Psychiatry* 143 : 1450, 1983.

Jouvent, R., Lecrubier, Y., Puech, A. J., et al. Antimanic effect of clonidine. *Am. J. Psychiatry* 137 : 1275, 1980.

Leckman, J. F., Hardin, M. T., and Riddle, M. A. Clonidine treatment of Gilles de la Tourette's Syndrome. *Arch. Gen. Psychiatry* 48 : 324, 1991.

San, L., Cami, J., Peir, J. M., et al. Efficacy of clonidine, guanfacine and methadone is the rapid detoxification of heroin addicts: A controlled clinical trial. *Br. J. Addict.* 85 : 141, 1990.

Zubenko, G. S., Cohen, B. M., Lipinski, J. F., and Jonas, J. M. Use of clonidine in treating neuroleptic-induced akathisia. *Psychiatry Res.* 13 : 253, 1984.

Zubenko, G. S., Cohen, B. M., Lipinski, J. F., and Jonas, J. M. Clonidine in the treatment of mania and mixed bipolar disorder. *Am. J. Psychiatry* 141 : 1617, 1984.

Verapamil

Barton, B. M., and Gitlin, M. J. Verapamil in treatment-resistant mania: An open trial. *J. Clin. Psychopharmacol.* 7 : 101, 1987.

Dubovsky, S. L., Franks, R. D., Lifschitz, M., and Cohen, P. Effectiveness of verapamil in the treatment of a manic patient. *Am. J. Psychiatry* 139 : 502, 1982.

Dubovsky, S. L., Franks, R. D., Allen, S., and Murphy, J. Calcium antagonists in mania: A double-blind study of verapamil. *Psychiatry Res.* 18 : 309, 1986.

Giannini, A. J., Houser, W. L., Loiselle, R. H., et al. Antimanic effects of verapamil. *Am. J. Psychiatry* 141 : 1602, 1984.

Gitlin, M., and Weiss, J. Verapamil as maintenance treatment in bipolar illness: A case report. *J. Clin. Psychopharmacol.* 4 : 341, 1984.

Disulfiram

Branchey, L., Davis, W., Lee, K. K., and Fuller, R. K. Psychiatric complications of disulfiram treatment. *Am. J. Psychiatry* 14 : 1310, 1987.

Eneanya, D. L., Bianchine, J. R., Duran, D. O., and Andresen, B. D. The actions and metabolic fate of disulfiram. *Ann. Rev. Pharmacol. Toxicol.* 21 : 575, 1981.

Fisher, C. M. Catatonia due to disulfiram toxicity. *Arch. Neurol.* 46 : 798, 1989.

Fuller, R. K., Branchey, L., Brightwell, D. R., et al. Disulfiram treatment of alcoholism: A Veterans Administration cooperative study. *J.A.M.A.* 256 : 1449, 1986.

Fuller, R. K., and Roth, H. P. Disulfiram for the treatment of alcoholism. *Ann. Intern. Med.* 90 : 901, 1979.

Kirubakaran, V., Liskow, B., Mayfield, D., and Faiman, M. D. Case report of acute disulfiram overdose. *Am. J. Psychiatry* 140 : 1513, 1983.

Sellers, E. M., Naranjo, C. A., and Peachey, J. E. Drugs to decrease alcohol consumption. *N. Engl. J. Med.* 305 : 1255, 1981.

Tacrine

Knapp, M. J., Knopman, D. S., Solomon, P. R., et al. A 30-week randomized controlled trial of high-dose tacrine in patients with Alzheimer's disease. *J.A.M.A.* 271 : 985, 1994.

Watkins, P. B., Zimmerman, H. J., Knapp, M. J., et al. Hepatotoxic effects of tacrine administration in patients with Alzheimer's disease. *J.A.M.A.* 271 : 992, 1994.

Index